Thai Spa Book

The Natural Asian Way to Health and Beauty

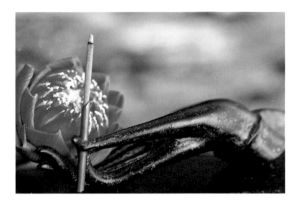

Chami Jotisalikorn
photos by Luca Invernizzi Tettoni

PERIPLUS

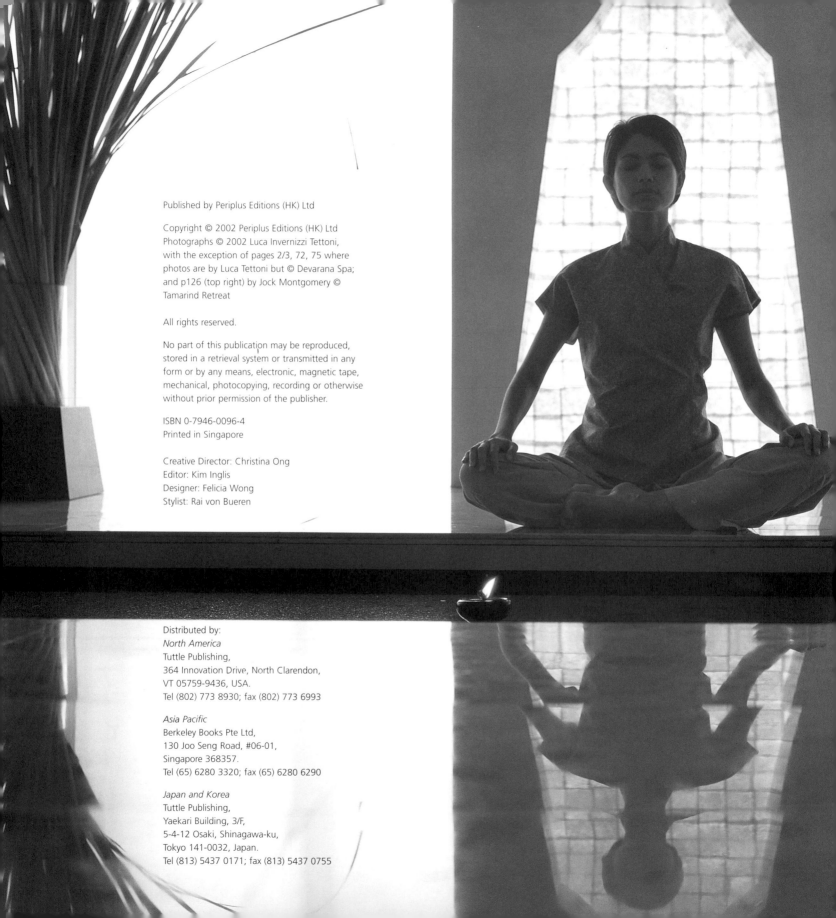

Published by Periplus Editions (HK) Ltd

ISBN 0-7946-0096-4
Printed in Singapore

Creative Director: Christina Ong
Editor: Kim Inglis
Designer: Felicia Wong
Stylist: Rai von Bueren

Distributed by:
North America
Tuttle Publishing,
364 Innovation Drive, North Clarendon,
VT 05759-9436, USA.
Tel (802) 773 8930; fax (802) 773 6993

Asia Pacific
Berkeley Books Pte Ltd,
130 Joo Seng Road, #06-01,
Singapore 368357.
Tel (65) 6280 3320; fax (65) 6280 6290

Japan and Korea
Tuttle Publishing,
Yaekari Building, 3/F,
5-4-12 Osaki, Shinagawa-ku,
Tokyo 141-0032, Japan.
Tel (813) 5437 0171; fax (813) 5437 0755

contents

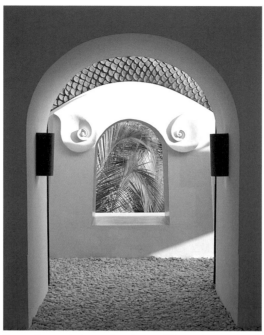

Elegant lines at the Lanna Spa, Regent Chiangmai Resort.

the thai spa experience

Thailand is the first choice retreat for well-travelled sybarites looking for stress-relief pampering — with silky smooth beaches and mouth-watering cuisine to boot. Everyone's heard of Thailand's famous spas, and the lucky ones have experienced their rejuvenating treatments, but what few realise is that the enticing menus at today's spas are formulated from ancient herbal healing traditions that have deep roots in Thai culture. Thai massage, for example, migrated from India with Buddhist monks and Brahmins in the 2nd and 3rd centuries BC; and the herbal heat compresses and Thai herbal steam are derived from folk medicine and ancient midwifery techniques.

The relaxing benefits of such blissful treatments are well known. But other than feeling fabulously indulged in the gentle hands of a soft-spoken Thai spa therapist, do these massages and herbal beauty therapies have real healing properties?

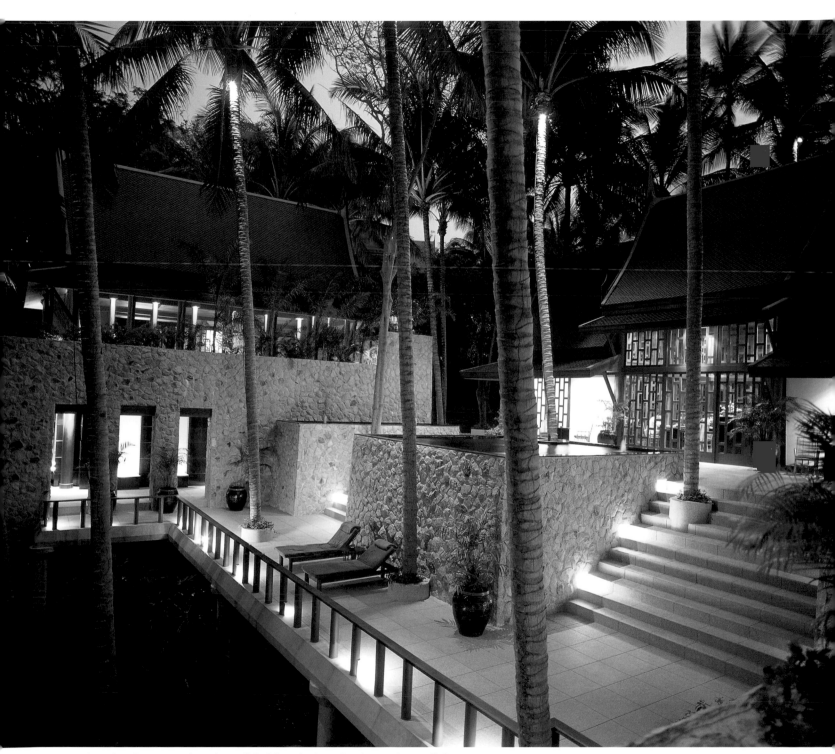

Teakwood pavilions come aglow when twilight falls at the Aman Spa, Amanpuri resort, Phuket.

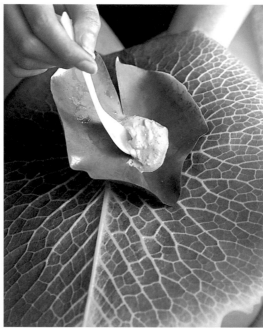

Turmeric paste is cherished by Thais for its skin healing properties
(above) while toning mask of cucumber (right) cools and revives.

The answer is a resounding 'yes'! The tradition of herbal healing in Thailand dates back for centuries; historical evidence suggests that the Thais practised an integrated system of medicine incorporating the Indian Ayurvedic system with Chinese practices, mixed with deep-rooted folk beliefs in the supernatural, mystical and astrological. The core philosophies of Thai medicine revolve around the balance among the four basic elements — earth, water, wind and fire — which comprise the essence of life, and appear as recurrent themes in many modern day spas.

Traditional massage and herbal remedies have cured the ailments of generations of Thais — that's why they're still in use today. And even if some scientists scoff at such techniques, says herbal therapist and owner of the Thai Herbal Spa, Khun Komon Chitprasert: "Once you experience the healing abilities yourself, your beliefs change".

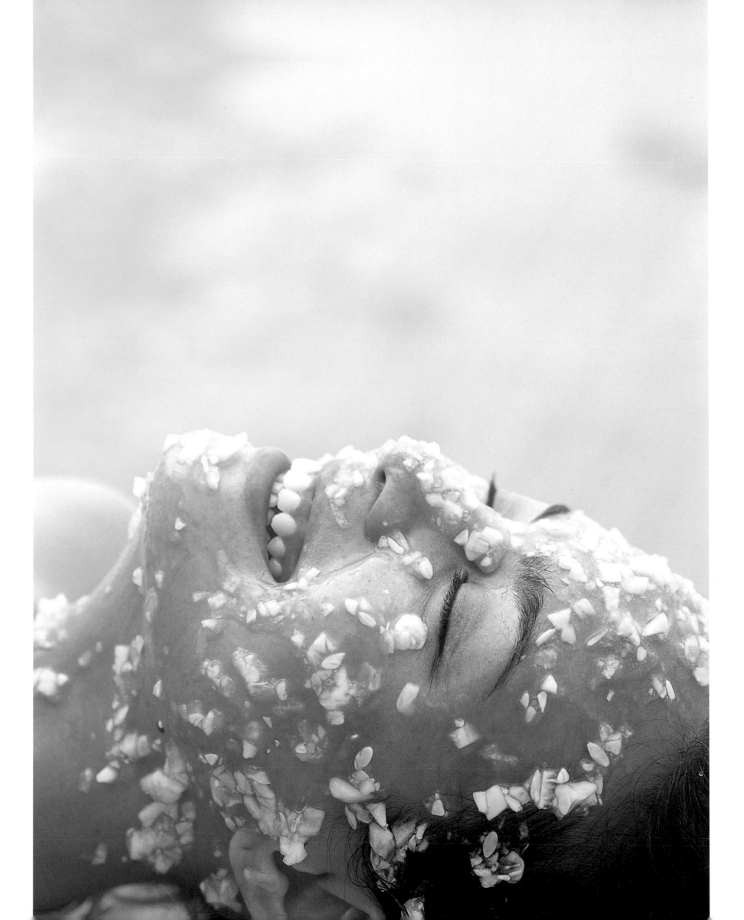

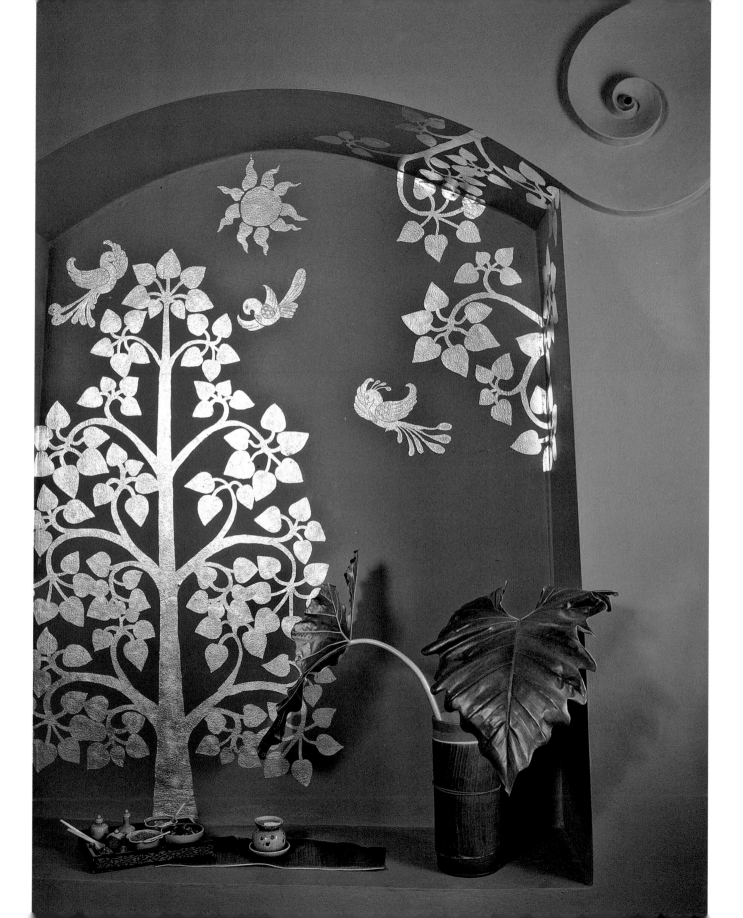

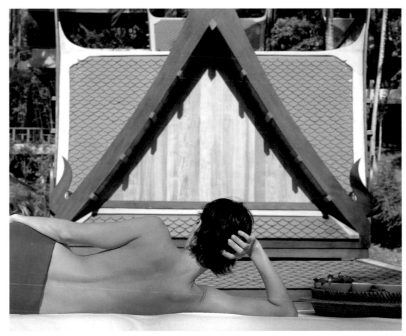

An outdoor treatment (above) fanned by cooling sea breezes at the Aman Spa.
Left: The Bodhi tree is a spiritual décor motif at the Lanna Spa.

In recent years, Thai traditional healing has experienced a revival, in part due to the efforts of Khun Pennapa Sapcharoen at the Institute of Thai Traditional Medicine; as a result, an interesting trend is the emergence of innovative new therapies based on ancient lore. For example, Bangkok's Nakriya House of Health and Beauty offers a unique fat and cellulite-reducing herbal bath and massage invented by owner Khun Shelida Buranasiri, derived from ancient midwifery practice. "Don't expect incense and candles," she warns, "my particular treatment is not about pampering, it's healing."

Her statement sums up the fundamental aspect of the Thai spa. The candles, flowers and luscious surroundings add to the sensory delights — but at the core of the best Thai spas is the Thai healing tradition, a special element offering the benefits of a glowing complexion, renewed energy and a feel-good factor, inside and out.

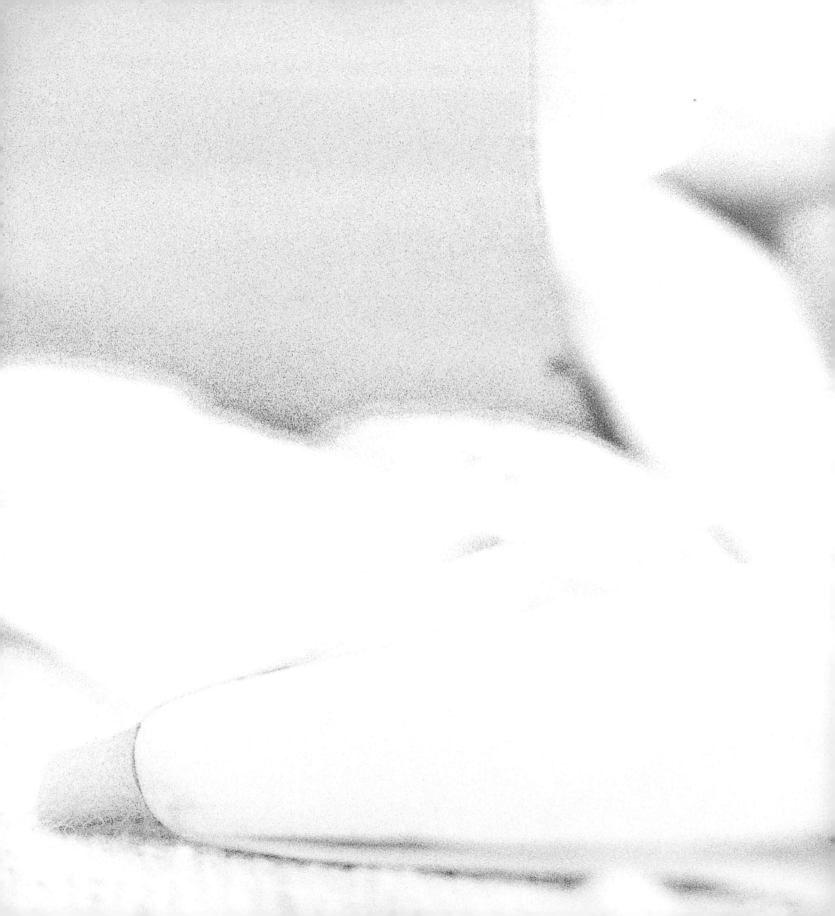

fragrant herbal healing

"Don't overlook the techniques of ancient remedies...the healing power of herbs and plants is far deeper and greater than what you only see on the surface."
— *Khun Komon Chitprasert, traditional herbal therapist and owner of Thai Herbal Spa*

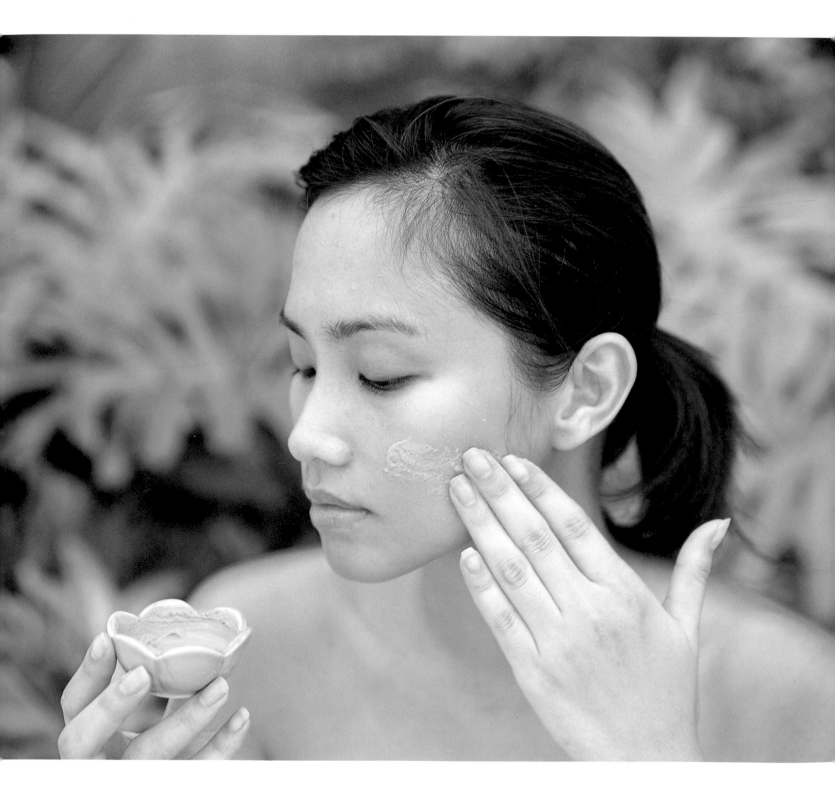

thai herbal

Traditional herbal remedies were once the secret domain of monks, local herbal healers and midwives. Because few people received a formal education in ancient times, healing traditions were passed down orally through generations within families. Very few records of healing knowledge exist; the ones that do are inscribed on manuscripts known as *samut khoi*, made of the same type of parchment used to record Buddhist scriptures.

Because much ancient medical knowledge came to Thailand from India through Buddhist monks, temples became the centres of learning with religious texts and manuscripts housed in special libraries. That is how monks gained a reputation as healers. There also existed a strong tradition of local folk medicine and herbal lore that involved animism, spirituality and astrology. Because monks themselves were folk people, some practices of folk medicine were incorporated into temple teachings. But as the vows of monkhood prohibited physical contact with women, midwives were trained in herbal medicine that specifically addressed issues of childbirth.

Local folk medicine contained elements of animism, such as the belief in the powers of rocks and stones for energy, and shamanism, with the concoction of medicines accompanied by chants and blessings. Midwifery was also concerned with the spiritual. An important element in midwifery was the belief that the midwife's role was to help prepare the spiritual path for the new baby that

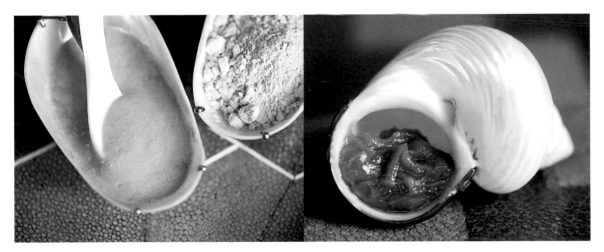

Opposite and left: Turmeric has long been used by Thais as a powerful skin soothing facial cosmetic. Fresh turmeric can irritate sensitive skins, so often a dried, powdered form is used in facial treatments.
Left: Yaa mong, or tiger balm, is a popular all-purpose remedy for insect bites, itchiness, rashes and skin irritations, and can come in herbal formulas such as this one.

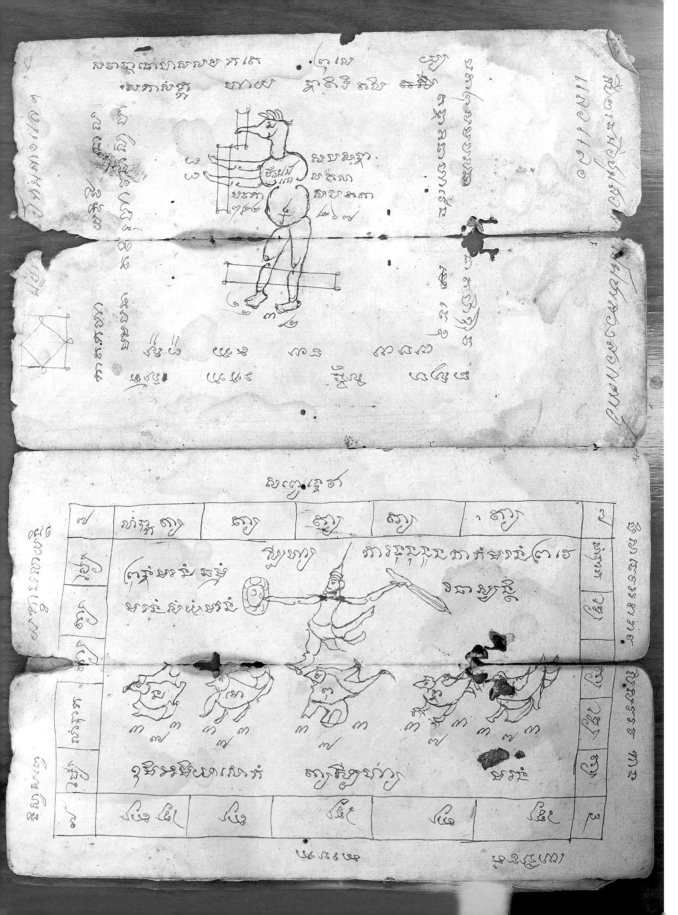

Left: Ancient Thai healing secrets were documented on parchment called *samut khoi*. This manuscript, in a northern Thai tribal dialect, describes herbal ingredients and remedies, as well as mystic beliefs and superstitions concerning the practice of traditional healing.

was about to enter the world. This was done by creating a state of utopia in the mind, body and spirit for the mother, through the practice of herbal cleansing rituals and massages.

There are many traditional beliefs governing the practice of herbal medicine, such as the regulation of the times and places for the collection of herbal ingredients. It is known that evening flowers such as jasmine and ylang-ylang are best collected at night, when their powers are most potent. Healers are required to perform certain chants while picking herbs; they ask forgiveness from mother earth, or Phra Mae Toranee, and receive her permission to gather the plants. The chants are accompanied by the lighting of incense. "The chants imbue the ingredients with greater healing powers than if you buy them from the market," says herbal therapist and owner of the Thai Herbal Spa in Bangkok, Khun Komon Chitprasert, who comes from a long line of healers from Phitsanulok in northern Thailand.

It is also said that certain plants must come from certain locations, due to the type and quality of soil. The soil for the *tong pan chang* plant, whose bark and flowers are used to treat internal injuries, is best in Sukhothai so the most effective ingredients are known to come from there. The time and date of plucking herbs is also crucial — at full moon is best because the energies of earth, moon and sun are at their most powerful then.

Thai herbs are often accompanied by stories of their healing properties. *Luuk blag mae*, or 'mother and daughter', is the name of a youth-enhancing herbal concoction that is said to make a mother look as young as her daughter. Legend has it that a mother who once ate the leaves of its ingredients immediately had fresher, younger skin! Another ingredient, the rhizome of *dog thong*, was used as a love potion for men because it was believed that it had the power to make girls fall in love.

According to traditional practitioners, herbal healing is a system of belief in the powers of nature and earth. "People are distracted by modern techniques and they overlook the power of ancient remedies," says Khun Komon. "They don't see how far-ranging the benefits of herbal medicine are. People should return to using traditional remedies, because their healing powers are far greater than what you only see on the surface."

Below left: Herbal cough syrup from the Chao Praya Abhaibhubejr hospital, Prachinburi province.
Below middle: Dried herbal ingredients and medicines are still sold in traditional medicine shops in Bangkok.
Below right: Some old remedies, such as these herbal breath-freshening tablets, remain popular to this day,

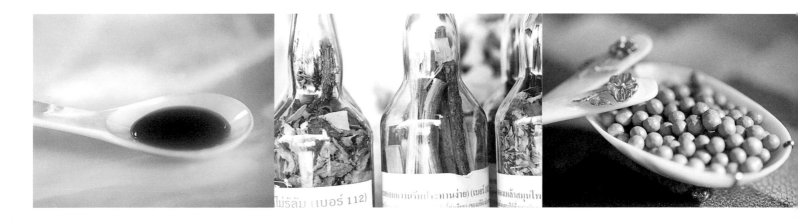

ไม่รั้ลืม (เบอร์ 112)

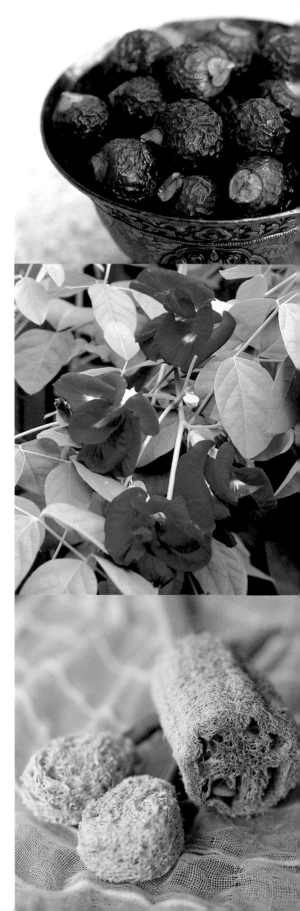

Clockwise from top left:

SOAP NUT (*Sapindus emarginatus*)
This ancient beauty ingredient derives its unusual name from the foam that is produced by crushing the fruit. For centuries Thai women have used the fruit to darken and thicken their hair. It is also believed to prevent hair loss.

KAFFIR LIME LEAF (*Citrus hystrix*)
Called *makrut* in Thai, this leaf is used in Thai cuisine to add a lemony flavour to soups and salads, while the zest is a popular ingredient in herbal compresses and the oil is used in aromatherapy. The fresh fruit is an all-purpose aid to hair beauty — making tresses soft and silky.

DEODORANT STONE
A rock-like mineral, *saan som* has been used by Thais as a natural deodorant and anti-perspirant for centuries. The 'stone' is wetted and then rubbed under the armpits. Before the advent of modern plumbing, the mineral was dropped into giant rainwater jars in order to 'deodorise' water; it drew sediment to the bottom of the jar, thus leaving the upper levels clear and fresh.

IVY GOURD LEAF (*Coccinia grandis*)
This attractive creeper is an age-old Thai medicinal ingredient used to soothe skin irritations, and is also a tasty ingredient in clear soups. Thais also found use for its moisturising properties as a beauty ingredient in body wraps and facial gels (it is good for use on normal skins.) The ripe fruit is high in vitamins, but its use is becoming rarer, because the fruit is tiny and difficult to find.

SEA SALT
Seen in glistening white heaps along the salt farms that dot Thailand's long coastal roads, natural sea salt has been adopted by many spas in beauty treatments. Mixed with essential oils, the gritty texture makes an effective body scrub.

LOOFAH (*Luffa cylindrica*)
Thais use the sweet-tasting young fruit of this gourd in a number of traditional dishes, and eat the flowers blanched, with chilli sauce. The dried mature fruit consists of thick fibres and is used as an exfoliating sponge in the bath.

BUTTERFLY PEA FLOWER (*Clitorea ternatea*)
For centuries Thai women have used the juices of *anchan*, a dark purple flower, to promote dark, lustrous, thick hair. It was also rubbed into babies' eyebrows to make the brows grow thick and long. The flower is rich in Bioflavinoid, an ingredient in modern-day hair products that stimulate hair growth.

COCONUT (*Cocos nucifera*)
The coconut has myriad uses in Thailand. When the fruit is ripe, the hard, white flesh is grated, soaked in water and squeezed to produce coconut milk, an important ingredient in Thai curries and desserts. The ripe fruit contains a juice that makes a refreshing drink in hot weather. Oil of copra, extracted from the dried meat, is used as an ingredient in the cosmetics industry. Coconut oil was used in the olden days to treat stiff joints; the oil was heated with *prai* (see page 19) and the mixture rubbed in.

RICE (*Oryza sativa*)
Rice is the lifeblood of Thai life. As the key crop and main food staple, it is highly revered in traditional culture and is protected by a goddess called Jao Mae Po Sob. The monarch officiates at the annual Royal Ploughing Ceremony, which marks the first day of the planting season. In the past Thais used rice to ward off ghosts — chanting monks endowed sacred properties onto rice that was then thrown on unwelcome spirits to chase them away. Many modern-day spas have adopted raw rice as an effective ingredient in natural body scrubs.

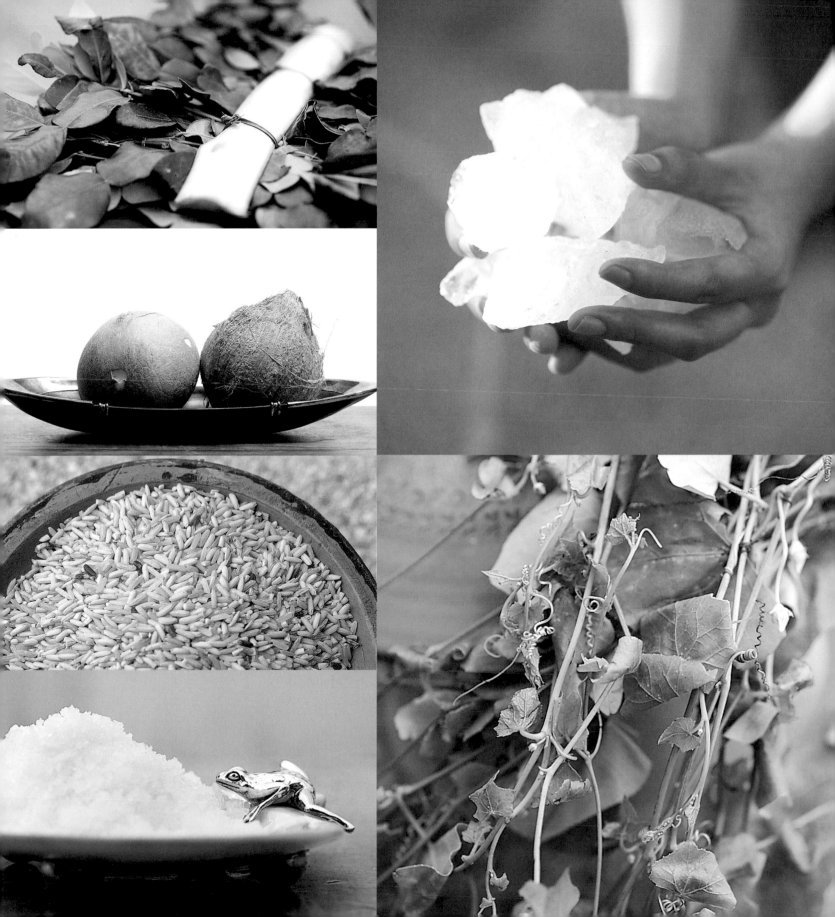

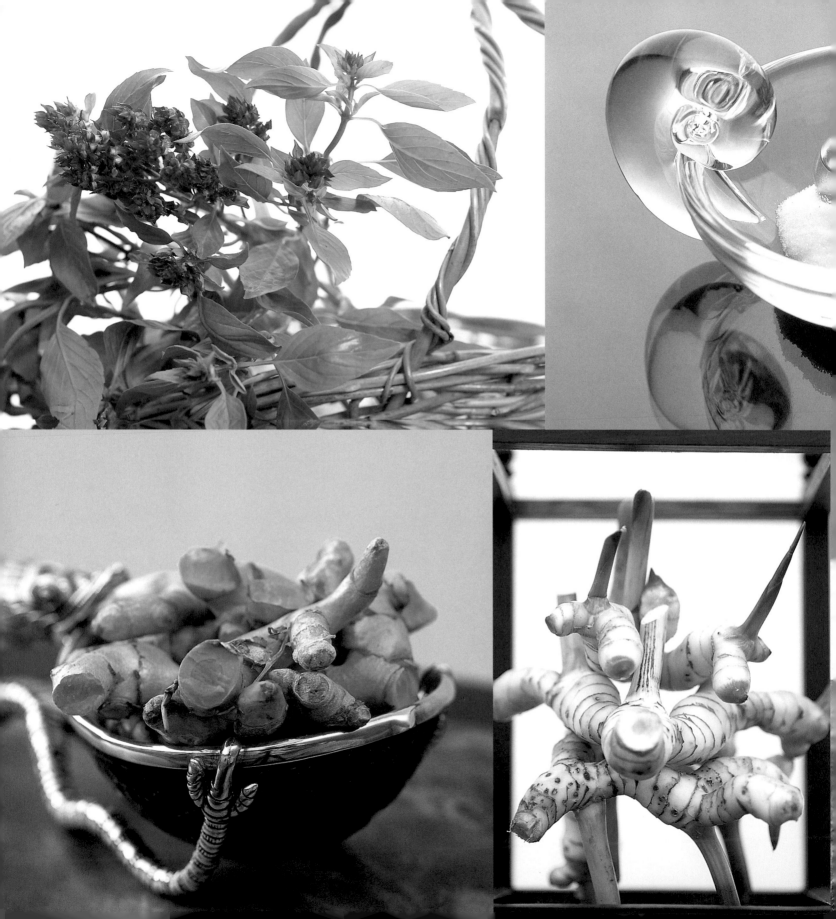

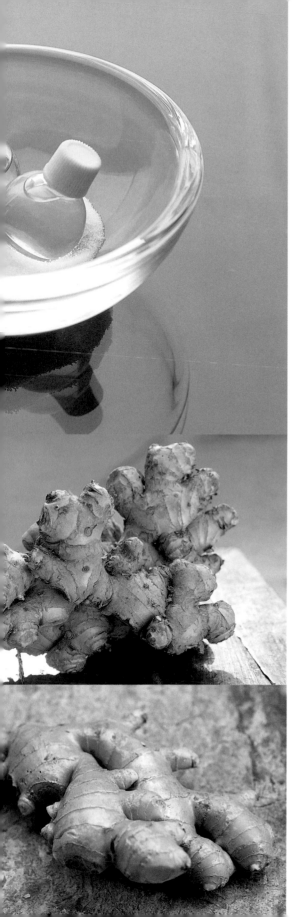

Clockwise from top left:

SWEET BASIL (*Ocimum basilicum*)

This fragrant, spicy herb — called *horapha* in Thai — is eaten raw or used as a flavouring in many local dishes. It has medicinal properties and is used in traditional healing to help reduce mucous in colds and flu, eliminate gas and aid digestion. As an aromatherapy ingredient, the essential oil of the basil plant is used to refresh the senses and relieve tiredness.

MENTHOL

Known as *phimsen* in Thai, this is a mineral with a sharp, minty smell similar to that of camphor. Its refreshing smell helps ease respiratory problems, coughs and blocked sinuses. *Phimsen* is an important ingredient in Thai traditional herbal steams.

PRAI (*Zingiber* sp)

Prai is a rhizome of the ginger family and has been used for centuries as a herbal ingredient in hot compresses that are applied to relieve muscular aches and pains. It is also a natural emollient and has been used by generations of Thai women to tone and soften the skin. *Prai* oil is also popular as a scalp conditioner and is used in aromatherapy.

GINGER (*Zingiber* sp)

Thais use both the young and mature ginger rhizome in many foods and beverages. Ginger is known as a stimulant that has a heating effect on the body. Taken as a herbal drink, it helps reduce gas and aids digestion. Traditionally, Thai mothers used a ginger treatment if their baby had an upset stomach. A paste of crushed ginger and rice liquor was rubbed on to the baby's tummy to soothe the stomach discomfort and reduce any gas. In aromatherapy, the essential oil is used to boost circulation and ease stiff muscles.

GALANGAL (*Languas galanga*)

This rhizome is often mistaken for ginger, but its whitish colour with a pinkish tinge identifies it as galangal, a popular ingredient in Thai soups and curries for its fragrant, tangy aroma. Though too pungent to be eaten raw, the fresh root is used in traditional medicine to relieve digestive ailments and cure skin diseases. Galangal finds its way into modern spa treatments as an ingredient in herbal body wraps.

TURMERIC (*Curcuma domestica*)

This orange-coloured rhizome is dried and crushed to form a powdered spice and colouring for many kinds of food. Called *khamin* in Thai, turmeric is one of the key ingredients in Thai healing concoctions. It is used in herbal medicine to treat stomach discomfort and in traditional cosmetics for skin care. When crushed, the oil the rhizome yields is an efficient natural moisturiser and it also has antiseptic properties.

Not pictured:

PAPAYA (*Carica papaya*)

The ripe fruit contains the enzyme papain, which is known for its digestive properties. The bright orange fruit contains large amounts of Vitamins A and C, and acts as a digestive when eaten unripe, or a laxative when eaten ripe. It is also known to contain AHA, making it a popular and effective ingredient in body wrap treatments to exfoliate and smoothe the skin.

THAI WHITE MUD (see page 101)

Thailand's famous white mud or *dinsaw pong* (the name means 'putted-up pencil' because it is a white chalk that expands in water) is a natural cooler. It has a pleasant smell and traditionally was used in the same manner as talcum powder after a shower, to help cool the body in hot weather. It is used as an ingredient in face masks and body wraps for its cooling properties.

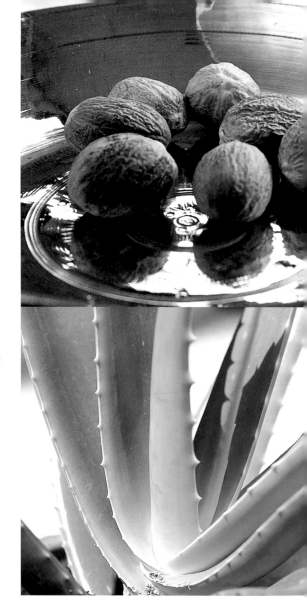

Clockwise from top left:

NUTMEG (*Myristica fragrans*)
Though not a commonly used ingredient in Thai cosmetics or cuisine, this spice has medicinal uses in southern Thailand. Here, the oil is extracted from ground nutmeg and is used in massage oil to soothe muscular aches and pains and stimulate the muscles. It has a warm, spicy scent that relieves fatigue.

LEMONGRASS (*Cymbopogon citratus*)
A signature ingredient in Thai cuisine, this grass-like herb has a sharp, fresh, lemony aroma, making it a favourite flavouring in food, drinks and cosmetics. As a medicinal herb, it was traditionally used to cure skin complaints and headaches, and was burnt to kill germs and repel insects. It is an ingredient in Thai herbal compresses for its soothing, invigorating and antiseptic properties, while the aroma relieves stress. As an ingredient in a traditional herbal steam bath, it helps clear the head and soothe hangovers.

MINT (*Mentha* sp)
Thais often add fresh mint to tangy salads; it is believed that mint aids digestion. In modern spa treatments it is used as an ingredient in body wraps and foot treatments for its refreshing smell. The essential oil of mint is used in aromatherapy to invigorate the senses and ease nasal congestion.

LIME (*Citrus* sp)
Lime is another signature ingredient in Thai cuisine: It is usually mixed with chilli and onions in soups and salads. As a spa ingredient, its acidity gives it the same qualities as tamarind (see photograph on right), but it is used in smaller quantities due to its small size. The essential oil is used in aromatherapy to boost circulation and it is an effective insect repellent. All citrus oils are also used as energisers.

TAMARIND (*Tamarindus indica*)
The incredibly sour tamarind fruit is eaten in a variety of ways in Thai cuisine and it also has a variety of medicinal uses: the bark is used as an astringent, the flowers can reduce blood pressure, and the fruit has a laxative effect. A refreshing tamarind drink can relieve constipation. The leaves are used in herbal steams as the acidity is thought to help the skin absorb the other herbal ingredients faster. Traditionally, wet tamarind was used as a beauty product: its high AHA content makes it an effective natural exfoliator and it was put on the face and body to brighten and smoothe the skin.

CAMPHOR (*Cinnamomum camphora*)
Extracted and processed from the camphor tree, *kalaboon* is a white powder-like substance with a cool, refreshingly minty smell used to ease and soothe respiration. The powder is used as an ingredient in Thai herbal baths and the leaves of the camphor tree are a vital ingredient in traditional herbal steams.

CUCUMBER (*Cucumis sativus*)
This crisp, refreshing vegetable has been used for hundreds of years as a face mask ingredient to help tone and moisturise the skin. Because of its high water content, chilled cucumber slices placed on the face provide immediate relief on a hot day.

ALOE VERA (*Aloe vera* syn. *Aloe barbadensis*)
Thais call this plant the 'crocodile tail plant' due to the appearance of its tapering, spiky leaves. When the leaves or stalks are pierced, a refreshing, healing gel oozes out. If applied to the skin, it soothes burns and is also a natural skin softener. Aloe gel is an effective natural sunburn soother and it is also good for moisturising dry or flaky skin.

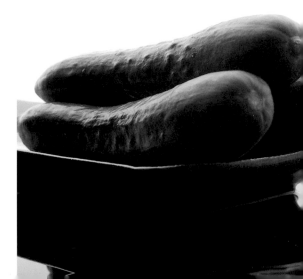

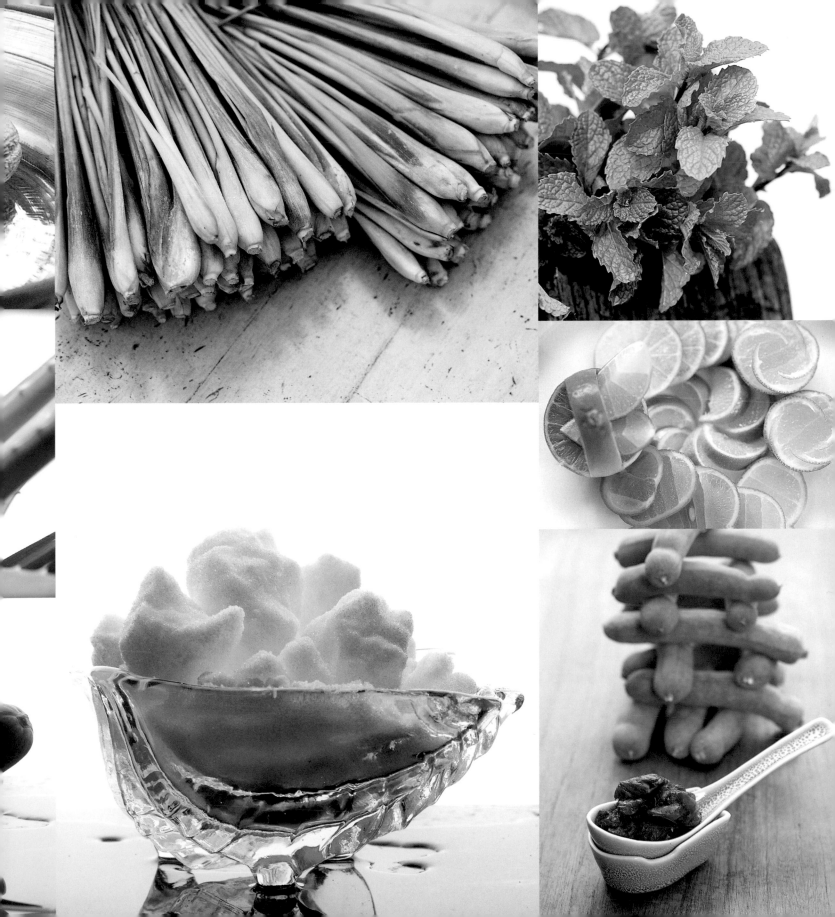

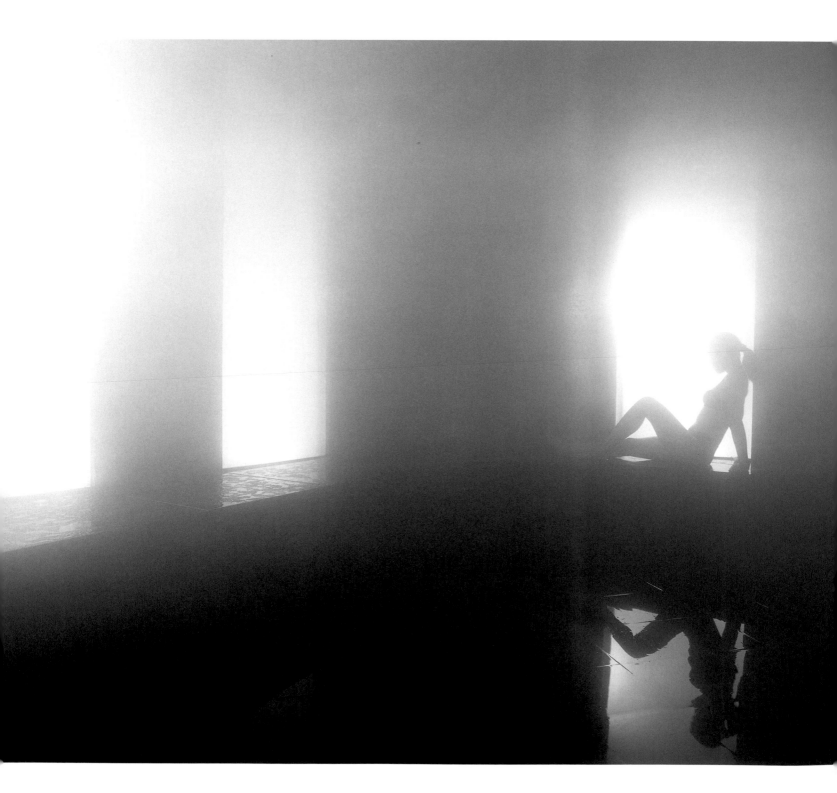

herbal heat

The unique Thai herbal steam is one of the best known of the traditional therapies. It traces its roots back to ancient times; formulae differ from region to region, as individual healers have their own recipes based on their own knowledge of local plants and their benefits. Furthermore, different healers have formulated specialised treatments to cure various health conditions.

What is common to all herbal steams, though, is that they have fantastic therapeutic effects on your body. All you do is step into a dreamy, misty, heavy-scented room, lie back, and let the steam vapours do their work. As they penetrate the skin's open pores and enter the lungs, the molecules from the medicinal herbs are absorbed into the body. It's a real vitality boost, and also helps you to relax and clears the head. A totally self-indulgent treat is to combine your herbal steam with a massage. The heat from the steam room warms and relaxes your muscles in preparation to be thoroughly stretched by the masseur. A herbal steam is also good before a body wrap, as ingredients put on the body will be more readily absorbed by steamed, softened skin.

Afficionados swear by the Tamarind Retreat steam on the island of Koh Samui. Built into a crevice between two boulders on the spa's hillside property, the cave-like steam room is a dreamy place to soothe the body and clear the head. Guests enjoy alternating warming bouts in the steam room with refreshing chilly dips in their cold plunge pool.

The numerous tamarind trees that are the spa's namesake provide plentiful leaves — one of the key ingredients in their herbal steam. Other ingredients include lemongrass for its antiseptic properties; *prai* to moisturise the skin, ease sprains or muscular pain; turmeric to relieve itching and cleanse wounds; camphor leaves for their respiratory benefits; Kaffir lime leaves and fruit to clear dandruff; beach morning glory to clear skin inflammations and allergies; and tamarind leaves to speed the absorption of herbal ingredients in the skin.

The folks at Tamarind Retreat claim that their steam treatment aids respiration, relieves sinusitis, bronchial asthma, general stuffiness and stimulates circulation. It is also good for aches and pains and it cleanses the skin's pores. Above all, it relaxes body and mind

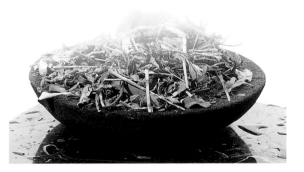

Opposite: The elegant lines of the black marble steam room at the Aman Spa, Amanpuri, Phuket provide an ultra-stylish setting for steam sessions. But the herbal steam comes with a word of warning: It isn't safe if you have hypertension or heart problems, and it's advisable to drink lots of water before, during and after the steam. *Left:* Ready-made preparations of dried ingredients can be bought in health stores around Thailand.

tangy citrus bathing

It's only one step from the traditional Thai steam therapy to the herbal bath, as many locally-grown herbs work well in water too. Inspired by the fabulous healing properties of Thai herbs and their ability to treat the body and revitalise the mind, the Banyan Tree Spa has come up with this herbal bath treatment to relax and cleanse your entire body. Here's how.

The ingredients used in this easy-to-make recipe can be found in any Thai kitchen — all you need is a piece of muslin cloth big enough to hold all the ingredients in a bundle.

Quarter cup	dried Kaffir lime peel
Quarter cup	dried ginger powder
Quarter cup	dried galangal
One cup	fresh pandanus leaves

Opposite: The popular herbal bath treatments offered in most Thai spas is a variation of the traditional herbal steam concept, and uses many of the same ingredients, such as lemongrass and Kaffir lime. *Right:* Thai Kaffir lime is inedible, but the fragrant fruit and leaves have medicinal properties used in body and hair treatments. The peel contains oil that softens and moisturises the skin when used in hot herbal baths.

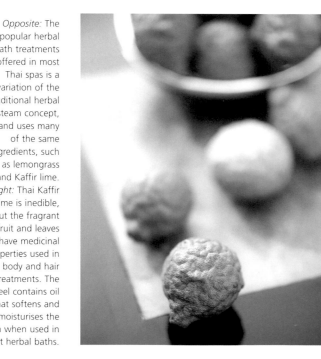

Using a mortar and pestle, crush the pandanus leaves well until the leaves become damp with their own juice. Mix all the ingredients together and wrap them into the muslin cloth to make a herbal pack. Tie the pack tightly with a cotton string.

Place the herbal pack under the running water so that the herbs soak in the water and fill the bathtub to the desired level. Shower and scrub your skin before stepping into the bath, then luxuriate in the scented water for 10–15 minutes. Afterwards, rinse off again under the shower and moisturise the skin with your favourite scented moisturising lotion.

Alternatively, you could try this traditional Thai steam with 3 or 4 Kaffir lime leaves, 2 tablespoons Kaffir lime zest, 2 slices *prai*, 6–8 stalks of sliced lemongrass, 1 sliced galangal root, a handful of tamarind leaves and 1 tablespoon camphor powder. Clean all the herbs and bring them to the boil in a rice cooker. When the steam starts to form, gently open the lid and sprinkle in the camphor powder and wait a few minutes. When more steam arises, sit opposite the cooker and cover yourself and the cooker with a blanket, all the while inhaling the aromatic vapours. Stay in your steam tent for 10–15 minutes. With repeated use, you'll notice a clearer complexion and less nasal congestion.

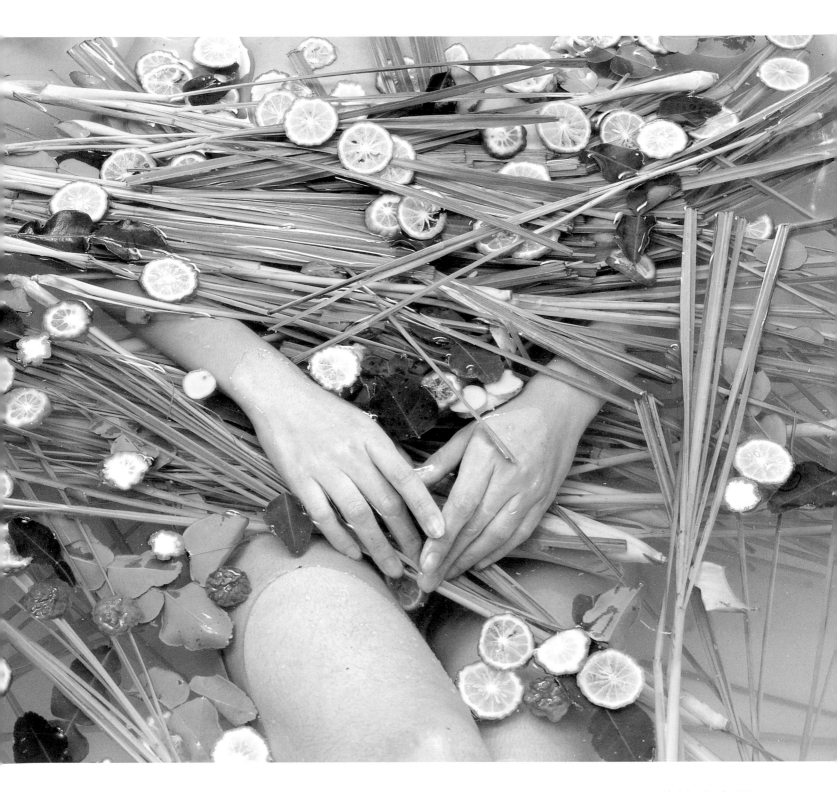

deep heat, thai-style

In Thailand, the round cotton bundles containing herbal mixtures were once the secret tools of ancient healers, and up until recently, could be obtained only from traditional healers or from the Thai massage school at Bangkok's Wat Po, or Temple of the Reclining Buddha. Nowadays, though, you can make your own with various combinations of herbs — for deep heat soothing of muscle aches and pains.

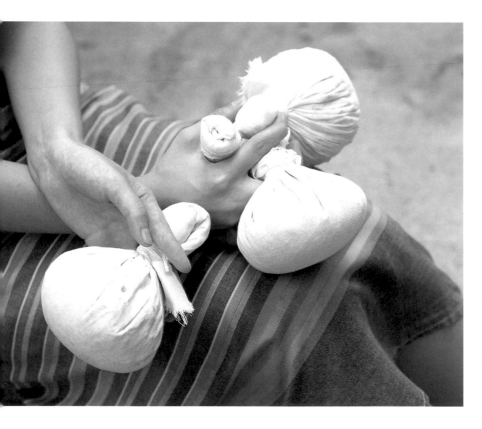

The origins of the Thai herbal heat compress are obscure, but it's known that such compresses were used to soothe the aching muscles of war-weary soldiers during the Thai-Burmese battles of the Ayutthaya period over 200 years ago. Such compresses were also popular in neighbouring Burma, Cambodia and Laos, though the formulae differ from region to region, depending on the local plants and herbs.

With the recent back-to-nature trend among stressed and health-conscious urbanites, these herbal compresses are now packaged and sold commercially in Bangkok's many health stores, so you can give yourself a quick-fix heat treatment at home. Some Thai women use these store-bought compresses on their abdomens after giving birth, to help ease the tired, bloated feeling that comes after childbirth. Called *prakop* in Thai, the herbal compress has been incorporated into modern spa treatments and is offered at a number of Thai spas, such as the Oriental Spa and the Banyan Tree Spa, often in conjunction with massage.

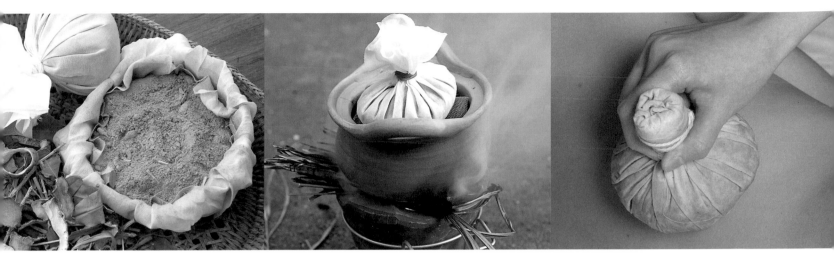

As with other herbal therapies, the ingredients in the compress may be mixed according to specific formulae to address specific ailments. Generally, the compress contains from 10 to 20 ingredients, though there are some standard ingredients that form the base of every compress.

The Oriental Spa in Bangkok has made waves with the way it combines traditional remedies with high-tech, modern techniques. It was the first Thai spa to incorporate this ancient healing method into their treatment menu, with their Oriental Herbal Pack treatment which combines massage therapy with the application of the herbal compress. If you want to make your own compress at home, they suggest you use some of the following healing ingredients:

Camphor: Its cooling and tingling sensation helps invigorate the skin.

Lemongrass: This has antiseptic properties to help clear up the skin.

Turmeric: Its antiseptic properties help soothe and cleanse irritated skin.

Prai: This ginger is a natural moisturiser that relieves muscular aches and pains while softening the skin.

Kaffir lime: These miracle limes help tone the skin.

Take a handful of each ingredient, and place them in a piece of cotton cloth and tie into a firm bundle. Heat the parcel over a steamer or hot pot before applying on to the body. Traditionally, the application was done in conjunction with massage — the sore muscles were worked first, then the heated compress was applied to the problem spots. The heat relaxes the aching muscles and helps to open the pores, allowing for better absorption of the herbal ingredients. Allow the heat to penetrate into your muscles, and feel stress and tension ease away beneath the healing kneading of a firm (but never painful) masseur.

Benefits include the soothing of sore and aching muscles, an easing of respiration with the ingredients camphor and menthol, and the reduction of tension through the heat and aromatic properties of the herbs.

Opposite: These herbal compresses have now become familiar sights in modern spas for relief of muscular aches and pains. *Above left:* Ready-made preparations, as either powdered or dried herbs, can be bought in Thai health stores. *Above centre:* Traditionally the bundle was steam-heated over a charcoal burner. Most spas today use an electric rice cooker for quick and easy steaming. *Above right:* Once heated, the compress is applied on sore muscles in conjunction with massage.

best for baby, best for mum

Herbal therapies devised by Thai midwives have long played a key role in Thai traditional healing. In the past, most births took place in the home, and women took advantage of the healing secrets that midwives passed down from one generation to the next. Here's how herbs can help a mother — before, during and after childbirth.

During pregnancy, most Thai women soothe the backaches and leg pains that come with bearing the weight of the child in the womb with Thai massage. And as antenatal care was supervised by a local midwife, she would mix herbal formulae for all the ailments associated with pregnancy and childbirth. Each mixture was customised to suit the individual patient, according to whether the patient's energy type was of the fire, water, earth, or wind element. Special ingredients, mainly herbal roots, bulbs and rhizomes, were used for post-pregnancy treatments. There are a number of rhizomes known to Thai healers for their benefits to the womb; most are identified by their specific healing properties, such as *waan chak mod luuk*, meaning 'womb-pulling rhizome', a large, bumpy root that is believed to help tighten the womb.

Most women would have been prescribed *yaa-hom*, or 'fragrant medicine'; this comes in the form of dusty gold pellets made from a blend of medicinal flowers and herbs including ylang-ylang, jasmine and camphor, the scent of which is inhaled to relieve feelings of nausea or morning sickness. The pellets may also be dissolved in water and drunk as a tonic to soothe feelings of faintness or dizziness.

During labour, a professional midwife was always on hand: her skills were in demand, and after the birth she would cut the umbilical cord with a sharpened bamboo stick. Known for its anti-bacterial properties, the bamboo stick didn't have to be sterilised; as well as being sharp and clean, it provided the added benefit of sterilising and cleansing the wound.

Immediately after giving birth, the new mother would undergo the famous *yuu fai* or 'staying with the fire' treatment for a period of three weeks. This intensive post-pregnancy sauna treatment was once so prevalent in Thai life that everyone has heard of it even though it is not often practised today. The treatment required the woman to lie in a room at home where a fire was kept burning in a charcoal stove at all times, thus creating an intensive sauna. The high temperature forced the body to sweat, thereby flushing out the toxins accumulated during pregnancy. The new mother was not allowed to bathe during this period, and the body was wiped down with a wet cloth instead. No herbs were used with the sauna, but *yuu fai* was supplemented by herbal treatments that helped reduce swelling and encouraged the womb and muscles get back into shape after the rigours of childbearing. Turmeric poultices were applied daily to the abdomen and buttocks, to help cleanse and tone the skin, bringing it back to health.

It was believed that, as well as ensuring complete recovery of the womb, the *yuu fai* treatment gave benefits in later life too. It was said that women who didn't undergo the sauna would become temperamental and experience mood swings upon reaching their 50s and 60s. And they would be more prone to aches and pains from during spells of cold or damp weather.

The new mother also took a daily herbal steam treatment using herbal mixtures specifically formulated for post-pregnant women. She sat in a small tent where medicinal herbs were steamed on a charcoal stove placed inside the tent. The treatment lasted about 10 to 20 minutes, and it was believed that the greater the amount of sweat, the better the detoxifying effects on the body.

As with other Thai herbal therapies, post-pregnancy healing treatments varied from region to region, with various ingredients and methods

of heat and herb applications. Khun Rungratree Kongwanyuen, Spa Manager at the Lanna Spa, remembers a post-pregnancy midwife therapy used by her older sister. Unique to their seaside hometown of Hua Hin, in Thailand's central Petchburi province, it was called *mod luuk khao ou* or 'womb returning into place'.

It consisted of a series of herbal incense sticks, the size and shape of cigars; each was composed of a special preparation of dried, crushed herbs that were mixed into a paste and moulded around a wick. Each stick was lit and then placed into a flat metal box called a *glong fai*. The metal boxes were in turn placed in a specially made, sectioned cotton belt resembling a money belt, tied around the new mother's waist. This heated belt was worn all day and night for 15 days; as each herbal incense stick burned out, it was replaced by a newly lit herbal stick. During this treatment, the new mother was able to go about her daily tasks as usual, without being confined to the tortures of a heated room, as in the *yuu fai* sauna method.

Below, left to right: Ingredients used in traditional midwife therapies include certain rhizomes that are known to have specific post-natal healing on the womb. The *yuu fai*, a herbal sauna treatment, requires the new mother to sit in a heated tent for a period of three weeks to cleanse the body of toxins accumulated during pregnancy.

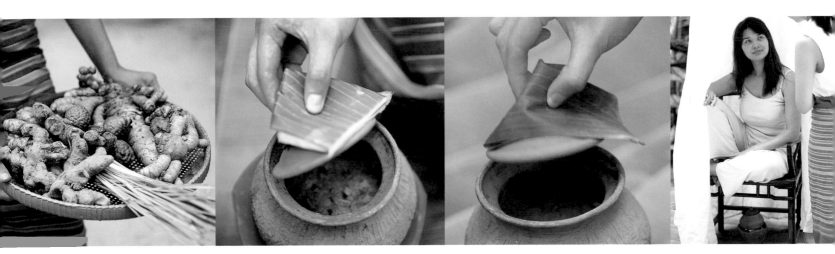

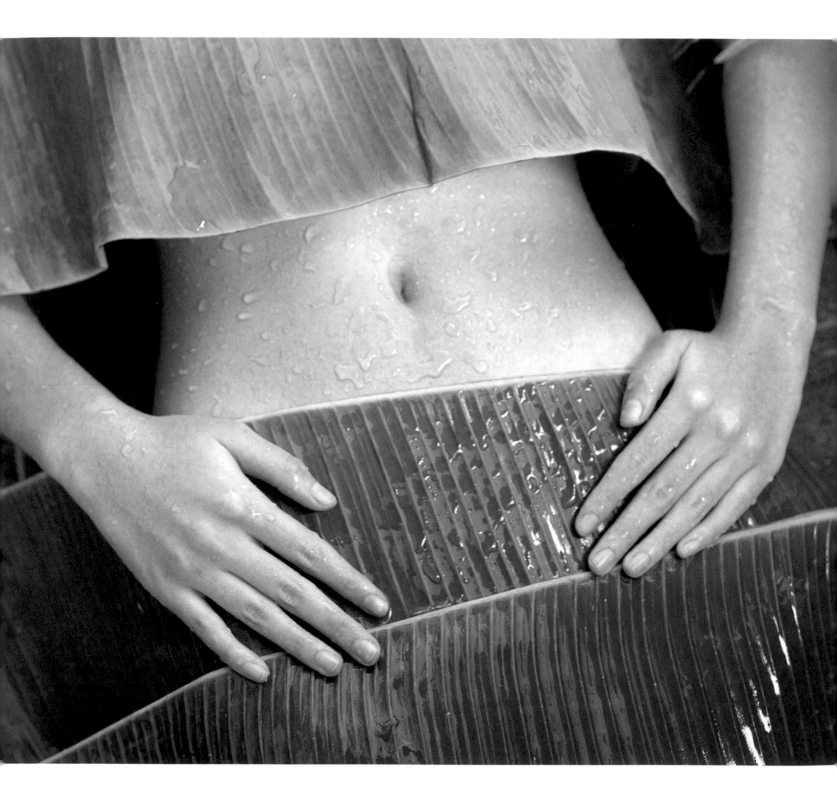

wrapping it up

Thai herbal practitioners have long recognised that the application of heat on the skin enhances the healing effects of herbs — hence the tradition of using herbal steams, saunas and heated compresses. Inspired by the age-old heat treatments used in Thai traditional medicine, modern-day spas have adapted this concept to create the Thai herbal body wrap.

First, you warm up in the herbal steam, then have a bracing body scrub to exfoliate dead surface skin, and finally a herbal mixture is massaged onto the entire body. You are then wrapped, mummy-like, in plastic and left cocooned under a blanket. Some spas may wrap you in a heated blanket to relax the muscles and induce sweat, while others use regular blankets whose natural warmth helps activate the heating effects of particular ingredients in the herbal mixture. As the body lies in the herbal wrap, the combination of heat and herbs takes effect —

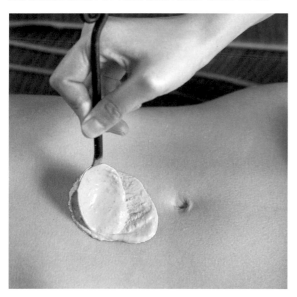

the heat helps open the pores, allowing for better absorption of the ingredients into the skin, and the herbal wrap works to detoxify, moisturise and soften the skin, depending on the particular mix of ingredients used.

Just as traditional healers had their own recipes for herbal remedies depending on their locality, the various Thai spas have their own versions of herbal body wraps that offer different therapeutic benefits. Bangkok's Oriental Spa harnesses natural ingredients that have been used in herbal healing for centuries in its Oriental Herbal Wrap Treatment. They use the following ingredients:

Thai White Mud (*dinsaw pong*) — helps draw out impurities, heals wounds, clears rashes

Turmeric — antibacterial skin freshener

Camphor — cleanses minor infections

Mint – antiseptic and antibacterial

Tamarind — contains vitamin C and calcium

Honey — heals and moisturises the skin

Milk — moisturises and softens the skin.

All the products are applied on the body and you're wrapped in plastic sheet. After 20 minutes it's washed off and the result is smoother, softened skin, with a healthy, radiant glow.

Opposite: The versatile banana leaf is put to myriad uses in Thai culture, from food wrappers to plates. Some Thai spas, such as the Lanna Spa at the Regent Chiangmai, use banana leaves as part of exotic herbal body wrap treatments.
Left: Healing turmeric root lends the distinctive yellow glow to the Oriental Herbal Wrap mixture shown here.

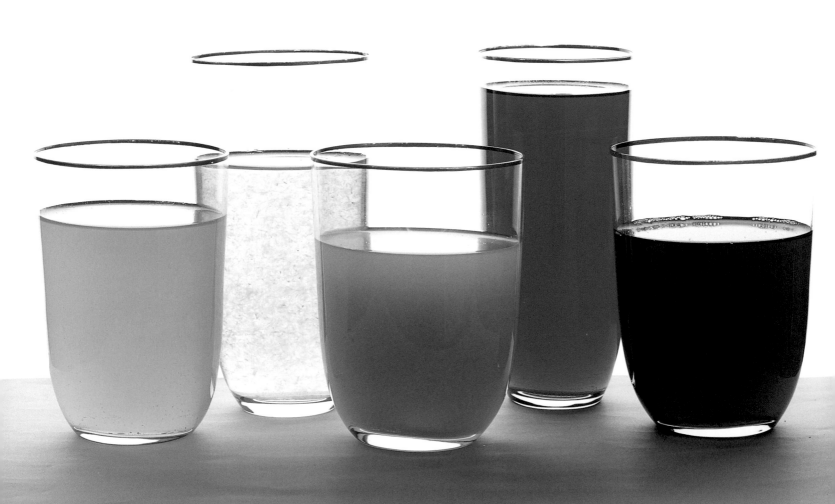

thai tonics

Looking good is not just a matter of what you put on the outside of your body; good looks come from within. A radiant complexion, healthy hair and skin and general well-being aren't the result of a beauty product or two. While it takes real will power to make radical changes in your diet, the easiest way to make a transition from unhealthy eating habits to a better new you is to start with what you drink.

The key to a good complexion is water — and plenty of it. Drinking lots of mineral water throughout the day not only makes you feel good, but keeps your skin hydrated and prevents it from looking parched. If you are watching your weight, a high water intake makes you feel less hungry. Try mixing a little fruit juice with mineral water and drink it half an hour before meals. Since your body takes 20 minutes to register feeling full, the juice will help cut your appetite by raising your blood sugar level.

Drink plenty of fresh fruit juices naturally rich in vitamins and minerals and avoid chemically concocted, artificially flavoured sodas. In a country abundant with luscious tropical fruits, Thais have been eating raw fruits and drinking fruit juices as part of their daily diet for centuries. And added to this is the age-old custom of drinking fresh herbal drinks and herbal infusions for their health benefits.

Thais have long drunk the fresh green juice of a herb called *bua bok*, or Asiatic pennywort (*Centella asiatica*). The sight of *bua bok* juice vendors ladling glasses of freshly pressed juice from carts piled high with fresh green herbs was once a common sight around Bangkok. The vitamin-rich juice relieves heartburn and many believe it aids the healing of

internal injuries if drunk immediately upon the appearance of bruises. The plant has astringent properties and in traditional herbal medicine it is applied topically to heal wounds and burns. Thais still drink it to remedy bruising and as a general health tonic, though these days the roadside vendors have all but vanished in the city.

Herbal infusions have had their place in the Thai diet for centuries. The number and variety of fruit, herb and vegetable drinks found in Thailand is comprehensive, with wide-ranging benefits for the health and complexion. Roselle, bael fruit, ginger, and lemongrass drinks are popular tonics and have a refreshing taste on hot days. Soy milk and chrysanthemum tea were brought into Thai culture by the Chinese immigrants, and now they have become part of the everyday Thai diet.

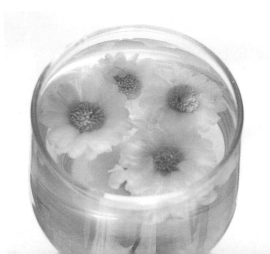

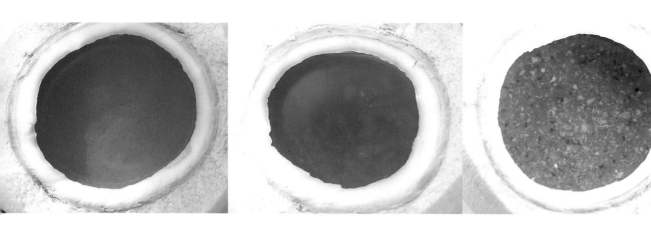

checks & balances

It's easy enough to make health drinks and tonics: choose your favourite fruits, roughly chop and throw them into a blender. See the benefits below. And for more details on some commonly used Thai ingredients, see the list opposite.

Fresh fruit drinks

Banana — rich in potassium, Vitamin B3, folic acid, calcium.

Coconut juice — helps flush the kidneys and bladder, removes toxins.

Guava — rich in Vitamin C.

Lime — high in Vitamin C.

Mango — high in calcium, magnesium, potassium.

Orange — high in Vitamin C.

Papaya — rich in Vitamins A and C, aids digestion.

Pineapple — high in calcium, magnesium, Vitamins C and B, aids digestion.

Pomelo — High in potassium and Vitamin C.

Star Fruit or Carambola — diuretic, relieves coughs.

Sugar Cane — high fructose content boosts energy, diuretic, eases coughs.

Tamarind — laxative effects help digestion.

Watermelon — diuretic, high water content quenches thirst while replenishing vitamins.

Fresh Herb and Vegetable Drinks

Aloe Vera — aids digestion, relieves peptic ulcers.

Asiatic pennywort — rich in Vitamin A, relieves heartburn, speeds the healing of bruises.

Pandanus — diuretic, the juice adds fragrance and colour to drinks.

Soy Milk — high in protein.

Herbal Infusions

Bael Fruit (*matoom*) — eases digestion.

Dried chrysanthemum — relieves heartburn.

Ginger — soothes upset stomachs, relieves nausea.

Lemongrass — diuretic, relieves gas.

Roselle (*grajiab*) — diuretic.

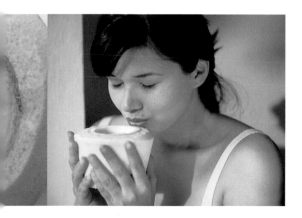

ROSELLE (*Hibiscus sabdariffa*)
A small shrub that grows in all parts of Thailand, the plant produces a deep red flower that contains a high amount of calcium and is used as a herbal diuretic health drink. It is believed to reduce fat levels in the blood, heal internal stomach wounds and improve circulation. Both the young leaves and young fruit are eaten in various Thai traditional dishes.

STAR FRUIT (*Averrhoa carambola*)
When cut horizontally, a slice of this juicy, crispy, yellowish fruit is star-shaped, hence the unusual name. It is also known as carambola, after its botanical name. It can have a slightly sour taste and when drunk as a juice is a refreshing thirst quencher in hot weather. The fruit also helps reduce blood sugar levels in diabetics.

DRIED CHRYSANTHEMUM FLOWER (*Chrysanthemum* sp)
This herbal health infusion is an example of how Chinese culinary traditions have been adopted into Thai culture because of the generations of Chinese immigrants that make up a fair percentage of the Thai population today. It is drunk as both a hot tea and an iced sweet drink, and is believed to reduce body heat and ease the intensity of heartburn.

SOYBEAN (*Glycine max*)
Soybean seeds contain more protein than any other legume, and are a good source of protein for vegetarians. After boiling, the beans can be eaten or used to make soymilk and other healthy drinks. Another legacy of the adoption of Chinese culture into Thai life, soy milk and soy curd are consumed in everyday cuisine.

MANGO (*Mangifera indica*)
There are a great variety of mangoes in Thailand and Thais eat them green, ripe, fresh, pickled, dry, and as snacks, savouries and desserts. In traditional medicine, the bark is used to cure dysentery, and the dried leaves treat diarrhoea. Mangoes are known to contain enzymes that help digest proteins, and therefore make a tasty and sweet ingredient in many health drinks.

PANDAN (*Pandanus amaryllifolius*)
A prominent ingredient in Thai cuisine, the long, leaves of this fragrant plant are a popular flavouring in desserts as well as steamed rice. The juice from the leaves is drunk as a refreshing hot weather pick-me-up. The whole plant is diuretic. As an ingredient in Thai herbal medicine, the roots are known for their anti-diabetic properties, and the leaves are used for treating skin diseases.

BAEL FRUIT (*Aegle marmelos*)
Though the raw fruit resembles a round ball, most Thais recognise *matoom*, as it is known in Thai, in its candied or dried version (see right) as it is rarely eaten fresh. Candied as a Thai dessert, bael fruit slices resemble horizontal cross sections of western tomatoes, with their reddish colour and radial sections. The unripe fruit has astringent and tonic properties, and the ripe fruit is a mild laxative. Though the fruit can be eaten raw, it is usually sliced and candied, or dried and drunk as a health drink.

ASIATIC PENNYWORT (*Centella asiatica*)
Called *bua bok* in Thai, this is a small creeping herb with pretty but bitter leaves that are very rich in Vitamin A. The juice has been drunk by Thais for centuries as a health drink for general well being, and as a herbal remedy for the healing of wounds and internal injuries. It is also used externally to accelerate the healing of burns and ulcerous skin ailments, and to help prevent scar formation.

BANANA (*Musa sp*)
The banana tree is found all over Thailand and the entire plant is used in many aspects of Thai life. The stem and fruit are used in Thai cuisine, and different parts of the tree have varying medicinal applications. The roots are diuretic, the sap from the stem is used as an astringent, and the blade of the leaves is used to stop bleeding. The unripe fruit is also an astringent, and the ripe banana is a laxative. Thais use the leaves in many practical applications, from everyday food wrappings to the intricately folded decorative containers used for food and festivals.

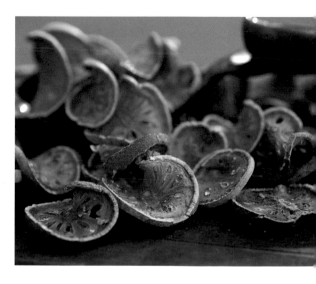

an appetite for health

In keeping with Thailand's tradition of drinking tonics, many Thai spas offer health drinks on their menus. Here they share some of their mouth-watering recipes, perfect for hot tropical days. Drink your way to optimum health.

Orange, Pepper and Alfalfa Juice (A Family Tonic)

This drink provides Vitamin C, beta carotene, potassium, and chlorophyll, all of which are important circulatory system nutrients that help ensure the health of your heart.

Ingredients (makes one glass)
1	large orange, peeled and chopped
1	medium red bell-pepper (capsicum), chopped
50 g	alfalfa sprouts
4	fresh cilantro (fresh coriander) springs with stems

Method
Process all the ingredients in a juice extractor. Mix well and serve.

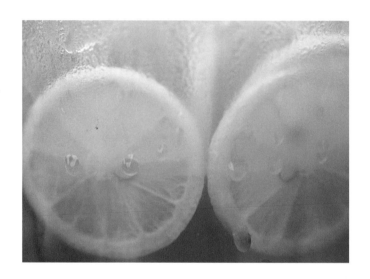

Guava, Apple and Chilli Juice (Back Pain Easer)

Guava is a source of Vitamin C, and chilli helps in depleting substance P in the sensory nerves. Turmeric is anti-inflammatory and oats provide micro-polysaccharides, which help increase the lubricating fluids in bone joints.

Ingredients (makes one glass)
½ cup	rolled oats
¼ cup (60 ml)	water
1	large guava, peeled and chopped
1	apple, chopped
1	serrano chilli, chopped
1 inch (2.5 cm)	fresh turmeric

Method
Combine oats and water, soak 15 minutes. Strain and squeeze the oats to extract all liquid, discard oats, reserving liquid. In a juice extractor, process remaining ingredients, then add to liquid. Mix well and serve.

Salad in a Glass (Blood Pressure Lifter)

Drinking this mineral-rich mix is just like drinking the equivalent of a salad. It is full of potassium, which helps in the regulation of blood pressure and can improve excessively low blood pressure.

Ingredients (makes one glass)
1	small cucumber, chopped
1	apple, chopped
1½	celery stalks with leaves, chopped
1	ripe tomato
¼ bunch	parsley

Process all ingredients in a juice extractor. Mix well and serve.

The recipes on this page courtesy of Le Royal Spa, Le Meridien Phuket Yacht Club.

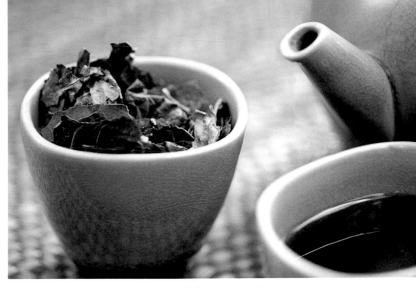

Herbal teas, introduced to Thailand from China, have now become an integral part of daily Thai life.

Aman Elixir

Guests at the Aman spa are greeted with a soothing herbal elixir (below) that is specially prepared according to a secret recipe. The elixir's main ingredient is white ginseng, a healing herb that stimulates the body to stave off illnesses such as digestive trouble and overcome fatigue. Cinnamon adds fragrance while purifying the blood and acting as a stimulant to expedite the function of other herbal ingredients. A cup of Aman Elixir helps your body reach a calming balance of yin and yang!

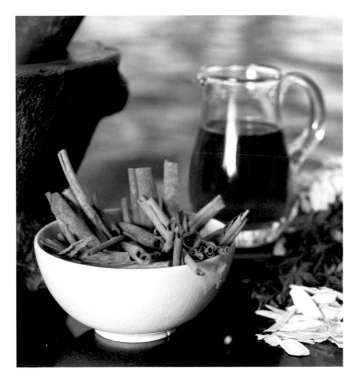

Reviving Fruit Combos
Pomelo, Pineapple and Mango Juice
— excellent for the digestive system and soothing for a nervous stomach.

Pomelo and Mango Juice
— a combination rich in calcium and magnesium.

Detox Spritz Cocktail
— pomelo, mango and sparkling mineral water cleanses the urinary system and helps rid the body of excess toxins.

Stress Buster Smoothie
— Banana, coconut milk and cinnamon are blended into a smoothie that soothes the nerves.

Recipes on this page courtesy of the Aman Spa, Amanpuri resort, Phuket.

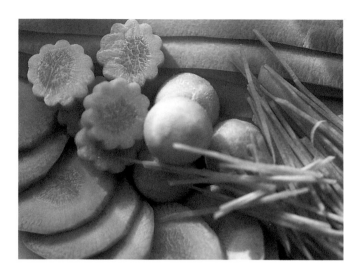

Carrot and Pineapple Juice

This bright orange drink is great for the digestion. Carrots are full of beta carotene, an important source of anti-oxidants, and naturally sweet Thai pineapple juice contains enzymes that help digest protein.

Ingredients (makes one pitcher)
2½ kg   fresh carrot, peeled and diced
2½ g   fresh pineapple, peeled and diced

Method
Mix the carrots and pinapple in a juice extractor to obtain approximately 2½ litres of juice. Serve chilled.

14 Fruits and Veg Drink

This comprehensive blend of fruits and veggies is bursting with vitamins and minerals to help get you energised and ready to face the day.

Ingredients (makes one pitcher)

2 stems	celery
6 leaves	cos lettuce
juice	from 4 fresh limes
1	banana
1	kiwi fruit
1½	green apple
7 cups	cold water
2	tomato
¼	onion
7 tablespoons	passionfruit juice
20	red seedless grapes
½	carrot
3 tablespoons	honey

Method
Mix all the ingredients in a blender and serve chilled.

Recipes on this page courtesy of Bangkok's Oriental Spa, where guests can choose from a selection of spa drinks, specially created from popular Thai herbs, fruits and vegetables.

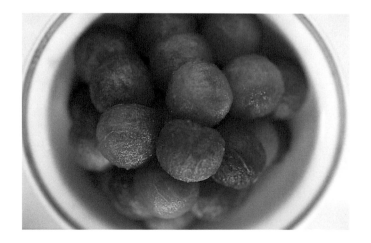

Roselle Juice

This beautiful red juice (see below) is made from the infusion of dried roselle flowers. Called *nam grajiab* in Thai, it is a popular Thai herbal drink taken to reduce body temperature and reduce fat in the blood. Its natural sour taste is sweetened with sugar syrup, and it makes a refreshing, healthy drink on a hot summer day.

Ingredients (makes one pitcher)

40 g	dried red roselle flowers
1 litre	water
200 g	sugar syrup

Method

Cover the roselle with water and boil and reduce until the juice is very red in colour. After boiling, add the sugar syrup and keep aside. To serve, mix 80 g juice with 20 g soda water and stir until well mixed. Serve chilled.

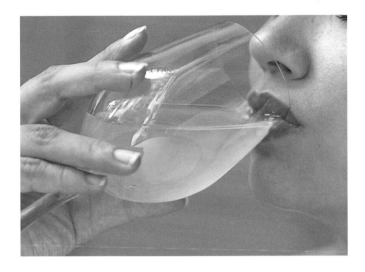

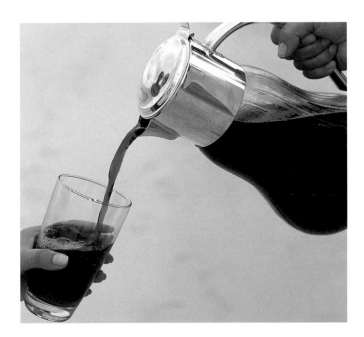

Aloe Vera and Pandanus Juice

These two ingredients make a bright green drink that is as healthy as it looks. Aloe vera juice is drunk by Thais as a holistic health drink to promote general well being, and the addition of pandanus leaf juice, a popular food colouring in Thai cuisine and desserts, gives the drink a refreshing colour and fragrance.

Ingredients (makes one pitcher)

500 g	aloe vera meat
1 litre	water
60 g	pandanus leaf juice
200 g	sugar syrup

Method

Cover the aloe vera with water. Bring the mixture to a boil and add the sugar syrup. Keep it chilled, then add the pandanus leaf juice to give a fresh green colour.

Recipes on this page ourtesy of Bangkok's Oriental Spa.

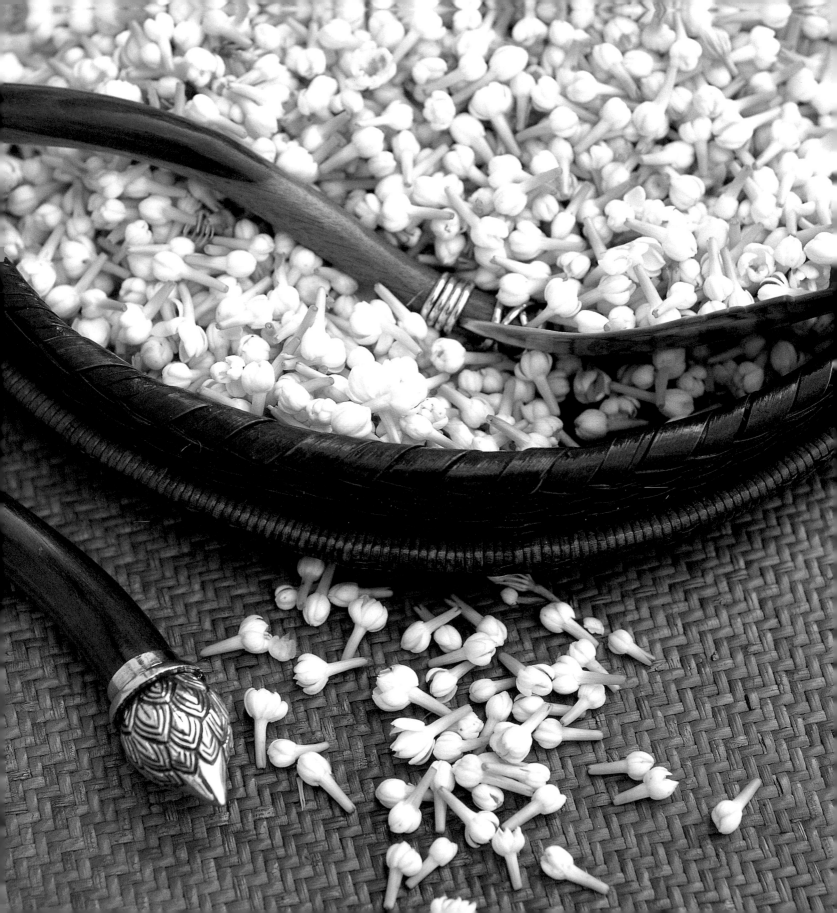

thai scents

One of the most recognisable smells in Thailand is the sweet fragrance of tropical flowers. Jasmine, champak, frangipani and orchids are used in decorative garlands and religious offerings in the daily rituals of Thai life, and their exotic, luxurious scents offer some of the most effectively relaxing essential oils that are used in aromatherapy massages.

The use of flower garlands is deeply rooted in Thai culture, and the tradition of garland making was a delicate and charming art that has been passed down from mother to daughter for centuries. Part of every young girl's education consisted of cultivating patience by sitting down quietly, stripping petals carefully off fresh flowers and learning how to make an exquisite garland. Jasmine is the main flower used in Thai garlands, with champak, red roses and purple orchids added for visual effect as well as to infuse subtle layers of aroma to the intricate floral weave.

From the small wrist-size strands for everyday use to the elaborate concoctions displayed at royal functions, garlands range in size and complexity of design. Seven-coloured garlands are the most favoured and expensive. For special occasions, such as weddings and going away parties, ribboned garlands are given as tokens of good wishes for future prosperity; these garlands are later given to a local temple in order to expedite a good marriage or a safe journey. Here, we examine some of Thailand's most favoured flowers and scents, and see how they are harnessed in treatments.

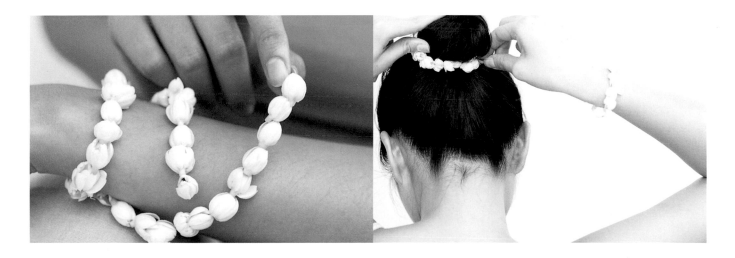

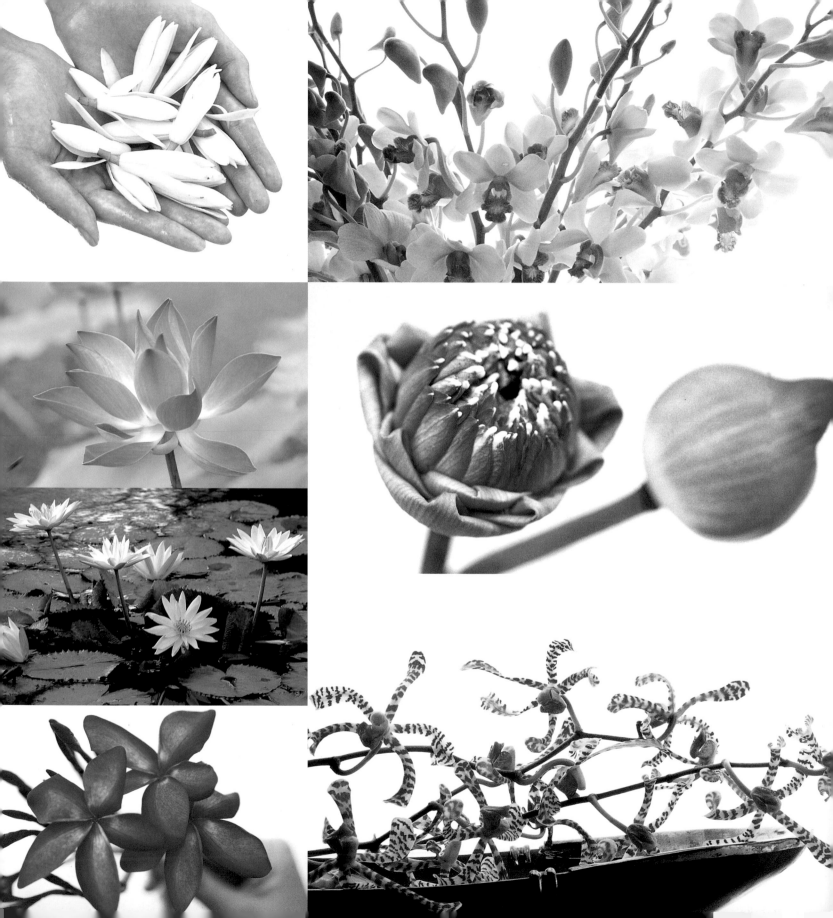

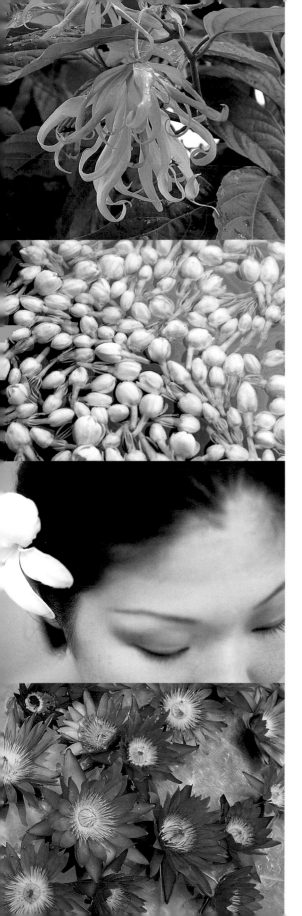

ORCHID (*Orchidaceae*)

A familiar symbol of Thailand, these exotic flowers grow profusely all over the country, in myriad colours, shapes and varieties. They are used in garlands and bouquets, and are often sprinkled in water jars as a decoration. They are also presented as small sprays as part of religious offerings.

LOTUS (*Nelumbo nucifera*)

The lotus flower has great religious significance in Thai culture. The entire plant is used in both food and medicine, and the blossom is a prevalent motif in Thai decoration as well. Significantly, the lotus is found growing in ditches and ponds all over Thailand, where society and culture revolves around water. The roots, young leaves, flower petals and seeds are eaten in traditional dishes. The leaves and petals are used as cigarette papers and wrappings for food, and the flowers are used in floral decorations and as religious offerings. Even the lotus seed hulls are used as a medium for growing mushrooms!

PLUMERIA or FRANGIPANI (*Plumeria* sp)

Found all over Thailand, especially in temples and in Buddhist monastery gardens, the frangipani tree was once considered taboo in Thai homes due to superstitious associations with its Thai name, *lantom*, which sounds like *ra-tom*, meaning sorrow — so the tree was thought to bring unhappiness. The beautifully sweet, fragrant blossoms are offered to Buddha either in garlands or on a plate, and worn by participants in traditional Thai festivals such as Songkran, or Thai New Year.

WATER LILY (*Nymphaea* sp)

This delightful aquatic flower is seen growing in ditches and ponds all over the county and is a popular decorative plant in homes and gardens. The blossoms come in white, yellow, and various shades of pink, purple and blue. Thai people eat the stalks raw and cooked, and the whole plant is used for decorative purposes.

YLANG-YLANG (*Cananga odorata*)

This exotic Asian flower is sweetly fragrant and produces an essential oil that is used in aromatherapy. It has a powerful, heavy, sensuous scent that is soothing and relaxing. In aromatherapy treatments, the perfume calms tension, lifts negative moods and increases sensuality. The flower was traditionally used as a medicinal ingredient in Asia to treat insect bites and inflamed skin, rejuvenate the hair, and ward off fever and infection.

CHAMPAK (*Michelia champaca*)

One of Thailand's many night-blooming flowers whose very powerful, sweet fragrance emerges most strongly after sunset, champak or *champee* flowers are used as religious offerings or in traditional Thai garlands. Their lovely smell makes them ideal ingredients to perfume rooms and the flowers have medicinal properties that help reduce body temperature and stimulate the heart.

JASMINE (*Jasminum* sp)

Jasmine flowers have great significance in Thailand and are made into garlands as decorations or offerings at religious ceremonies. Their pure white colour and delightfully fragrant aroma make them an ideal token for showing respect to Buddha or to monks. As a cuisine ingredient, the flowers are soaked in water to release a fragrant smell, which is then used to flavour desserts. As a traditional herbal remedy, jasmine was believed to help children with chicken-pox. The crushed flower was mixed with rice water, then put in the bath to reduce the itchiness. It was also made into a drink to help cure the disease.

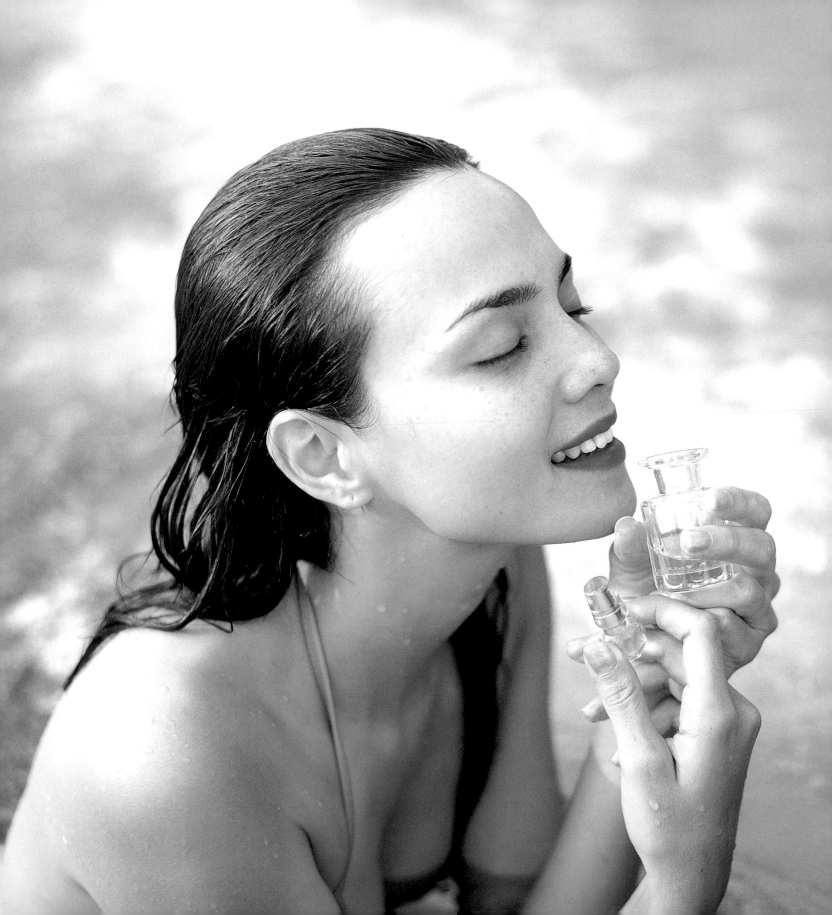

thai secrets of sensual healing

Healing through scent is an ancient tradition and the Thais have long believed in the powerful properties of perfume. They harness the fragrance of Thai flowers in a number of innovative ways; check out these aromatic ideas.

The traditional *yaa-hom* is a mix of herbs and flowers, whose key ingredients include refreshing menthol, sensuous ylang-ylang, sweet jasmine and champak blossoms. It's believed that a whiff of this herbal medicine can treat faintness, cure dizziness, soothe headaches, banish nausea and relieve gas. There's also a modern-day version in the form of the commercially marketed sniffing tube called *yaa-dom*, or 'smelling medicine'. The size of a lipstick, *yaa-dom* contains either oil of camphor, or a mix of camphor and menthol. When inhaled, it helps with dizziness or faintness, and is also handy in providing relief from unpleasant odours. Vastly popular among modern young Thais, its use reflects the age-old habit of using aromatic herbal remedies.

So how can the smell of herbs and flowers heal our frazzled nerves? Through aromatherapy, a healing practice that dates back to ancient times. that's how. By harnessing the fragrance of essential oils from plants, aromatherapy triggers the senses and affects our emotional and physical states. A plant's aroma comes from its essential oils, which contain dozens of complex chemicals that have the ability to effect reactions in our nervous systems, thus affecting our moods. The oil molecules are so minute and evaporate so quickly that they can penetrate human skin and enter the bloodstream and organs. As very few substances can penetrate skin, this makes essential oils uniquely therapeutic.

Here, we consider some of the essential oils commonly used in Thailand, their applications, and give you some tips for a variety of feel-good uses and blends. But however you use them, the end results are the same — you'll feel calm, relaxed, refreshed — all through the power of scent.

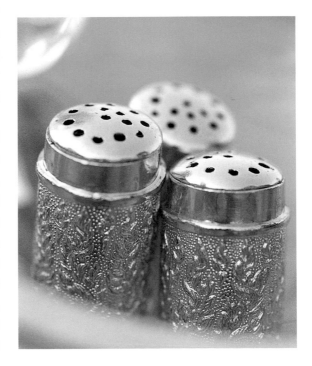

Left: All Thais keep a bottle of traditional *yaa-hom* or 'fragrant medicine' in their medicine cabinet, to be inhaled as a quick-fix remedy for various everyday ailments.

fragrant herbal: thai essential oils

Essential oils are derived from different parts of various plants. They come from petals, roots, rinds, stalks, seeds, sap, nuts, leaves or bark, depending on the plant's unique aromatic properties. Jasmine essential oil comes from the flower petals, and because the scent of this flower is most concentrated at night when the flowers are one day old, they need to be hand picked before dawn to obtain the best oil. Also, different oils can come from a single plant. For example, the orange tree produces three oils — neroli from the blossoms, petitgrain from the leaves, and orange oil from the fruit's zest. Each is an individual oil with its own properties.

Aromas from essential oils can soothe a headache, lull you to sleep, speed healing and calm nervous tension. Whether you realise it or not, you're affected by these essential oils every day — when you cut a lime, its essential oil squirts out and instantly evaporates into the air, releasing a tangy, sharp, citrus smell that has a refreshing effect.

The following oils are derived from traditional Thai herbs and flowers. All are familiar aromas in Thai cuisine and healing treatments. They can be used alone, or combined for different effects. Try some, or all, of them. Their sweet, spicy, sensuous, tangy and invigorating scents are guaranteed to recreate the bliss of a tropical Thai spa.

Opposite and right: Keeping oils for home use is an easy way to pamper yourself. Storing your oils in artistic containers, such as these bottles from Lotus Arts de Vivre, adds a luxurious touch to any bathroom or dressing table.

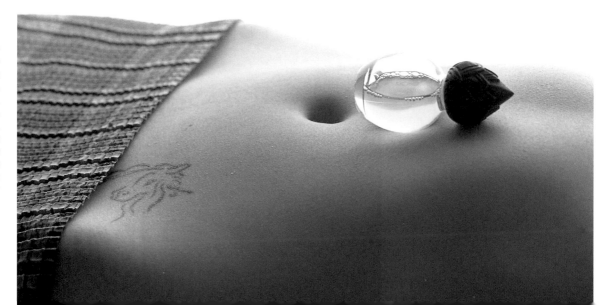

BASIL
- The essential oil is extracted from flowering sweet basil (*Ocimum basilicum*) and has a warm, spicy-sweet smell with a high concentration of camphor that is refreshing, light and uplifting.
- It is used for nervous insomnia, anxiety, fatigue, insect bites, headaches, poor circulation and muscular aches or sprains. A few drops on a tissue clears the head. It can be diluted with massage oil, rubbed into the skin to relieve insect bites or aches and pains.
- Basil should be avoided during pregnancy. It is potent and can be irritating on some skin types.

CAMPHOR
- The oil is extracted from the wood, root stump and young branches of the camphor tree (*Cinnamomum camphora*) and is known for its sharp, refreshingly minty, pungent fumes.
- It is good for muscular aches and sprains. Camphor can be used in massage but its scent is potent and it should be well diluted for massaging directly onto aching tissue. A few drops in a cotton ball or on curtain hems can make a good insect repellent.

CITRONELLA
- The oil is extracted from freshly dried citronella grass (*Cymbopogon nardus*) and has a strong, lemony smell.
- Citronella leaves were traditionally used as poultices for fever, pain and to speed healing. The essential oil is a strong antiseptic and air deodorant. It is renowned throughout Asia as an insect repellent.
- Applying the diluted oil directly on mosquito or other insect bites will stop the itching and act as an antiseptic.
- It should be avoided by pregnant women

CLOVE
- The essential oil is extracted from the leaves and dried clove buds and has a strong, woody, sweet smell.
- It was used by the Chinese as a breath freshener and in other cultures of the world was worn in ornaments around the neck to ward off disease. It is also an age-old remedy for toothache. Oil of clove is anti-bacterial and warms the skin and reduces swelling.
- It is used in massage to warm the skin, reduce swelling, and provide temporary relief from arthritis, rheumatism, sprains and bruises. Massaged on the abdomen, it relieves gastritis and stomach upset. One drop added to a half glass of water can be gargled to freshen the breath and ease sore throats.
- Its warm, spicy scent is used in aromatherapy to relax the mind and relieve fatigue.

EUCALYPTUS
- The oil is extracted from the twigs and leaves of the eucalyptus tree (*Eucalyptus* sp) and has a stimulating smell that clears the head and has a cooling effect on the skin.
- It is an excellent decongestant for flu and colds. It soothes muscular aches and pains and helps heal abrasions. A few drops in an oil burner will disinfect a room and ease your breathing at night. It can

be used in a chest massage, in a hot bath, or as a hot chest poultice.
- It can be diluted into a carrier oil and massaged into aching muscles for soothing effect.

GINGER
- Ginger (*Zingiber officinale*) has been used in food and medicines since ancient times. It was traditionally recommended for stomach ailments and its warming effect helps bring down a fever.
- The oil is extracted from the dried rhizome of the ginger plant and has a sharp, tangy, spicy smell with warming, stimulating, astringent and antiseptic properties.
- It is good for boosting the circulation, relieving coughs, stomach aches, muscle stiffness, or exhaustion. The smell is good for clearing the head and energising the body. It is effective in a bath or massage for its warming, soothing effect.

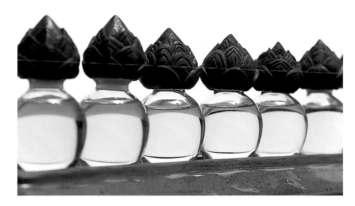

JASMINE
- The oil is extracted from one-day-old jasmine flowers that must be hand-picked before dawn, which accounts for its high price. Jasmine (*Jasminum officinale*) is cherished for its romantic, sensuous, sweet scent and is a much-used ingredient in toiletries and perfumes.
- The smell is relaxing and uplifting and is excellent for relieving depression, stress, fatigue, irritablity and pre-menstrual syndrome. A few drops in an oil burner will make you feel relaxed and sensuous.

LEMONGRASS
- Lemongrass was a traditional remedy for skin complaints and was burned to kill germs. It is now mainly used to flavour foods, drinks and toiletries.
- The oil is extracted from the fresh or dried *Cymbopogon citratus* plant and has a strong lemony smell that is soothing, healing, invigorating, antiseptic and deodorising.
- It is useful for treating headaches, poor circulation, and as an insect repellent. If it is well diluted and massaged directly onto irritated skin, it will boost the circulation and speed healing. Used in a steam bath, it clears the head and cures hangovers.

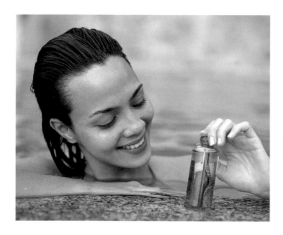
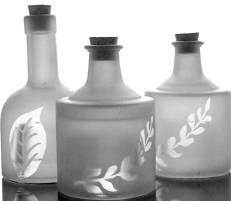
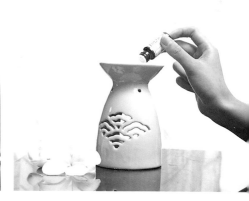

LIME
• The oil is extracted from the peel of the fruit (*Citrus aurantifolia*). It has a sharp, sweet citrus smell and is antiseptic and stimulating.
• It is used for greasy skin, varicose veins, poor circulation, cellulite, respiratory problems, colds, flu, fever, or infection. It makes a soothing warm bath, and can be applied as a poultice for breathing problems.
• Lime essential oil should be applied moderately and may irritate the skin, especially when exposed to sunshine after application. It has a short shelf life, so it should be used within six months to a year of purchase.

PEPPERMINT
• The oil is extracted from the fresh or semi-dried leaves and flowers of this herb (*Mentha x piperata*). The essential oil is nearly one-third menthol, which is why it invigorates, stimulates, and is soothing, refreshing and cooling.
• It is excellent for headaches, mental fatigue, muscular pain, sunburn, insect bites, nausea, indigestion and pre-menstrual syndrome.
• Peppermint essential oil is very potent and must always be diluted before applying on the skin or before going to sleep. It should always be used in moderation.

MANDARIN
• The essential oil is extracted from the peel of the ripe mandarin orange fruit (*Citrus reticulata*).and has a sweet, orange smell that has a sedative, calming effect.
• It is used to heal stretch marks, scars, and to relieve fluid retention and stress, and eases irritability, insomnia, restlessness and nervous tension. It is good in massage, baths and inhalation. It makes a wonderful massage for the buttocks, hips and thighs, as it helps reduce stretch marks.
• Mandarin essential oil may irritate the skin, especially if exposed to sunlight after application. It should be used in moderation.

NUTMEG
• The essential oil is extracted from the seeds of *Myristica fragrans* through steam distillation and its warm, spicy aroma relieves fatigue, relieves stress and lowers anxiety.
• This is a medicinal oil that is anti-inflammatory and has a gently warming effect, which is why it is used in the south of Thailand to relieve muscular pains and sore joints.
• The warm, comforting aroma is emotionally invigorating and stimulating. It is also used to treat nausea, vomiting and indigestion.
• It is very potent and could be toxic if used incorrectly. It should be used in very small amounts with a carrier oil.
• It should never be used in bath water, during pregnancy or while lactating. It should never be used on children or the elderly.

TANGERINE
• The oil is extracted from the fresh fruit peel of the fruit *Citrus reticulata*, and has a sweet, tangy, citrus fragrance and is a striking orange colour.
• The oil has mild stimulating properties and its gentle, calming effect makes it suitable for children and the elderly. It is especially useful in massage blends to tone the skin, and help heal scars and stretch marks. The aroma has a soothing effect that relieves stress and nervousness, and induces relaxation. It is an uplifting aroma that induces positive feelings while encouraging tranquility.
• It should never be taken internally, and strong sunlight should be avoided after using this oil.

YLANG-YLANG
• The oil is extracted from the freshly picked flower (*Cananga odorata*) and has a sweet, strong floral smell that is sensual and relaxing on the mind and emotions, rather than on muscular pains.
• It is one of the best oils for calming tension, lifting negative moods and increasing sensuality. A few drops in a massage oil will soothe stress, improve the mood and stimulate the senses.
• It is very potent and should always be used in moderation and diluted before application.

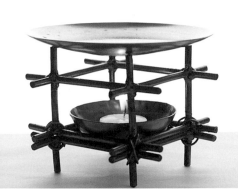

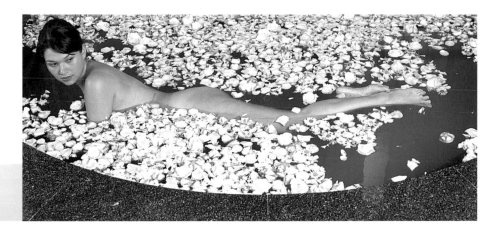

aromatic ideas

BATHS

The most relaxing way to use essential oils is to add them to your bath — you only need to use a few drops of oil. The steam and warmth evaporate the oils and intensify the aroma, while the water softens the skin and speeds up oil absorption.

BEAUTY TREATMENTS

Some essential oils have properties that can soothe and heal skin, rejuvenate complexions, reduce oiliness, and some just have a good smell. They make effective cleansers, masks, and moisturisers, which make you look and feel good.

BODY MOISTURISERS

Essential oils penetrate the skin so quickly and deeply that they make excellent and inexpensive body moisturisers. You can make your own by adding a few drops to a rich carrier oil, or to any simple unscented body moisturising lotion.

FOOTBATHS

Make a relaxing footbath by adding a few drops of essential oil to a basin of water and then soaking your feet. The oils refresh tired feet, soothe aches or help reduce perspiration.

HOT POULTICES

Essential oils applied with heat are a great way to relieve muscular pains and reduce chest congestion. Add a few drops of essential oil to a bowl of very hot water. Wearing rubber gloves, dip flannel or small towel into the bowl, squeeze out the excess water and place it over the affected area until it has cooled. Repeat the process.

MASSAGE

Massage combines the senses of touch and smell, as the essential oils are diluted in a carrier oil and rubbed directly onto the skin. Massage has the added benefit of stimulating the circulation, enabling the oils to disperse rapidly around the body. For more details of massage, see pages 50–51.

OIL BURNERS

Oil burners provide a way to warm essential oils so that their aroma diffuses across a room. They are little ceramic pots with a candle at the bottom and a saucer on top holding water in which a few drops of essential oil are added. The candle heats the water and the oil vaporises into the air.

POTPOURRI

To make your own potpourri, mix a few drops of essential oils and add to a bowl of dried flowers, herbs, leaves or seed pods. Cover the bowl for a while, then toss and stir the mixture so that it absorbs the aromas. The potpourri will scent your room for a few weeks.

ROOM SPRAYS

You can make your own therapeutic air fresheners using your favourite fragrances by mixing a few drops of essential oil with water in a pump spray. Shake well, then spray the room.

SLEEP TREATMENTS

A few drops of your favourite oil added to a tissue by your bed will not only help lull you to a relaxing sleep, but you'll continue to benefit from the aromatic effects as you inhale it while you sleep.

Opposite: Rubbing oils directly on to the skin is highly therapeutic, as it combines massage with aromatherapy. Storing home oils in artistic containers such as these from Lotus Arts de Vivre, adds a luxurious touch to any room. A convenient aromatherapy kit from Mandara Spa consisting of an oil burner, essential oil and two candles. *Above left:* An aromatic oil burner, such as this from the Lanna Spa, can be a stylish as well as effective way to diffuse scents through the home. *Above right:* A few drops of essential oil in a hot tub intensifies the aroma, giving you the oil's full therapeutic effects.

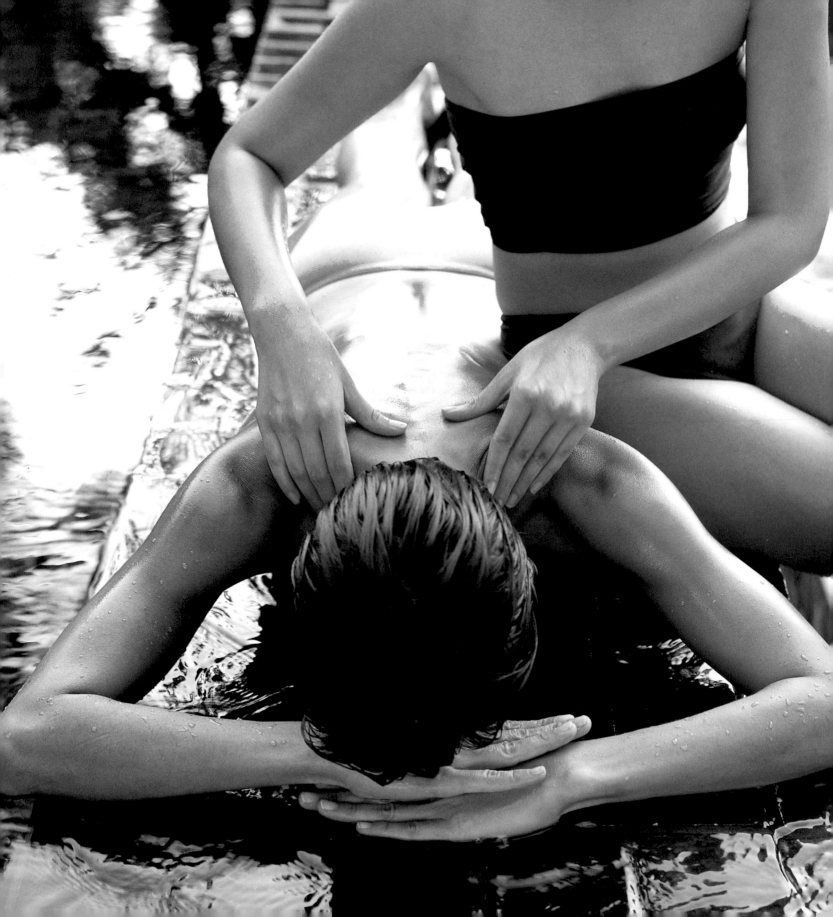

rites of massage

A good massage is always welcome relief to tired and aching muscles. But add the scents of essential oils and you get the heady aromas and extra healing benefits of aromatherapy. Here are some tips for using essential oils correctly.

Essential oils are very potent and highly concentrated, so should only rarely be used in their undiluted form. They are very volatile, that is, they evaporate quickly on contact with air. This is why they work so quickly, but it also means they need to be stored in airtight bottles. Ultraviolet light destroys essential oils, so they need to be kept in opaque (dark brown or blue) bottles and kept away from direct sunlight.

Never apply essential oils directly onto the skin, and never take them internally. They should only be used in drops; some essential oils are so potent they can even be toxic when misused. Oils must always be diluted in a plain carrier oil for massage (15–20 drops in 60 ml or 12 tsp carrier oil; 7–10 drops in 30 ml or 6 tsp carrier oil; 3–5 drops in 15 ml or 3 tsp carrier oil), or in water for a bath (use 8–10 drops maximum in one bath).

The best carrier oils to mix with essential oils are pure, cold pressed plant oils, because they help spread the essential oils evenly, slow down the evaporation rate, and increase the absorption into the skin. Mineral oils, such as baby oil, don't penetrate well into the skin, so are not good carriers. The best carrier oils for body massage are grapeseed, sweet almond, sunflower, safflower, peanut, soybean and sesame.

Many spas create their own oil blends. Some can be bought and taken home, such as the Mandara Spa's line of aromatic massage oils. Try these:

• Mandara Aromatherapy Oil (Romantic)
A blend of of sandalwood, patchouli and ylang-ylang to soothe the nervous system, nourish the skin and promote new skin growth.

• **Harmony Aromatherapy Oil (Balancing)**
A refreshing blend of bergamot, lavender, ylang-ylang and mandarin to calm the nervous system, while gently refreshing the senses.

• **Tranquility Aromatherapy Oil (Calming)**
A relaxing blend of vetiver, ylang-ylang and lavender that soothes the body and calms the mind. A highly beneficial blend for anyone suffering from insomnia, stress, emotional anxiety or jet lag.

• **Thailand Spice Aromatherapy Oil (Energizing)**
A spicy and aromatic blend of ginger, cloves, lemongrass and cinnamon that results in an exotic, tropical bouquet that helps to stimulate and warm the body.

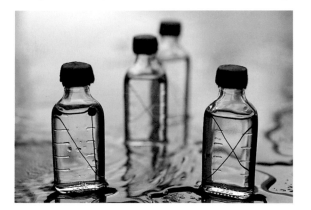

Left: The Mandara Spa's Mandara Oil for romance, Harmony Oil for balancing, Tranquility Oil for calming, and Thailand Spice Oil for energizing.

thai scents and sensibilities

Many everyday aches and pains can be helped by the soothing power of scent. In addition to their exotic fragrances, many essential oils have healing, anti-bacterial and anti-viral properties. Here we give a list of some common complaints and how they can be helped by Thai essential oils.

Acne: Lemongrass is effective on oily, problem skin because it is anti-bacterial, antiseptic and healing.

Backache: Camphor, citronella or eucalyptus are relaxing and have a warming effect that soothes muscular pain.

Circulation: Basil, ginger, lemongrass, peppermint, ylang-ylang and lime help boost the blood flow if you don't exercise enough or stand up too long.

Colds and Coughs: Peppermint, eucalyptus, lime, camphor and ginger are soothing when inhaled to relieve congestion and coughs.

Depression: Ylang-ylang, jasmine and bergamot can be relaxing and uplifting when you are feeling lethargic, miserable and gloomy.

Fatigue and stress: Eucalyptus, lemongrass, peppermint, ginger, basil, bergamot, jasmine or tangerine can relax and rejuvenate your mind and body when you are exhausted or stressed.

Hangover: Peppermint or lemongrass helps clear the head, energise the senses, and reduce nausea after a night of too much alcohol.

Headache: Eucalyptus, peppermint or lemongrass can help clear the head when used in inhalation or with a gentle head massage.

Insect bites: Peppermint, basil or citronella are anti-inflammatory, antiseptic and soothing, and effective for treating swelling, itchiness and inflammation.

Insect repellent: Camphor, lemongrass, citronella or basil can be dropped on your clothing or curtains to make natural, fragrant, non-toxic insecticides.

Insomnia: Basil, jasmine, or ylang-ylang drops in a warm bath are calming, and can help you relax before going to bed.

Jetlag: Peppermint clears the head, while orange is refreshing and relaxing, easing the disorientation and exhaustion that can result after a long flight.

Nausea: Peppermint, lime or ginger inhaled in a tissue can help relieve nausea resulting from dizziness, bad food or motion sickness.

Pre-Menstrual Syndrome: Bergamot, peppermint or jasmine lift your mood, and help with the moodiness or depression that can accompany menstruation.

Opposite: Steam inhalation is a classic method of aromatherapy, and is a popular way to ease colds and congestion. A few drops of peppermint, camphor, eucalyptus or lime in a bowl of steaming water will help clear stuffy heads and add a glow to your face in no time!

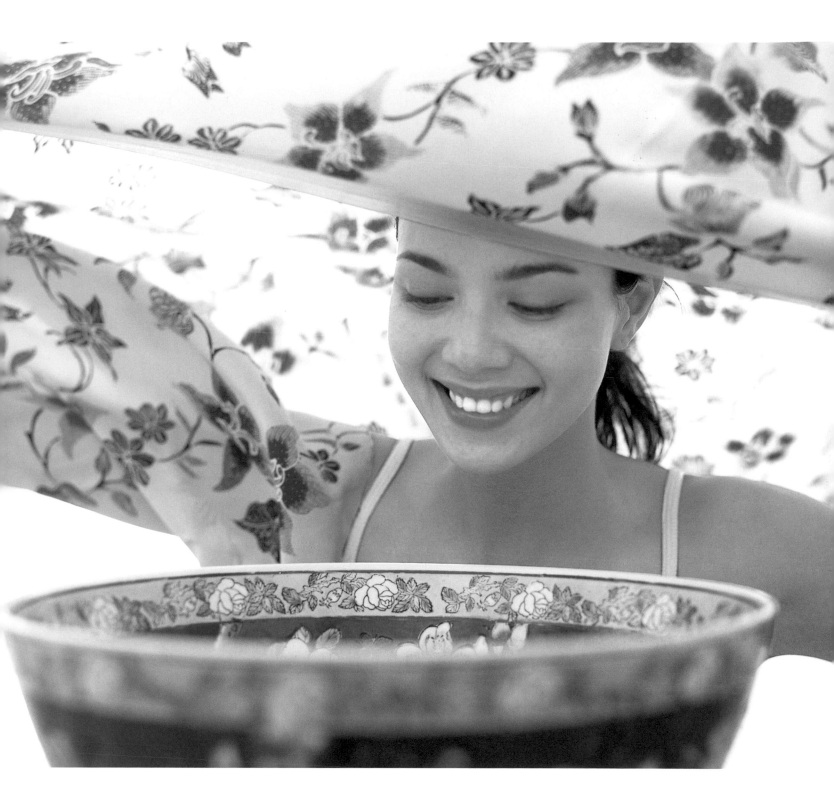

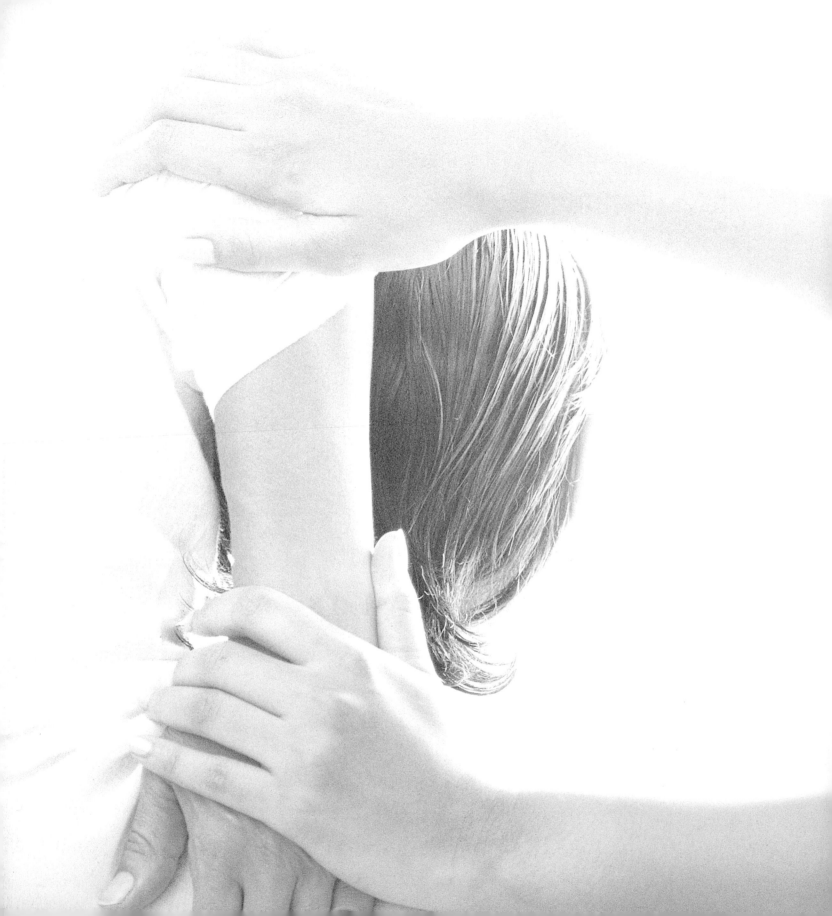

the power of touch

"No matter what you call a treatment or where it is given, no matter what ingredients, oils or essences you use — the most natural, pure and healing thing in the world is a caring touch."
— *Ian Bell, spa manager, The Aman Spa*

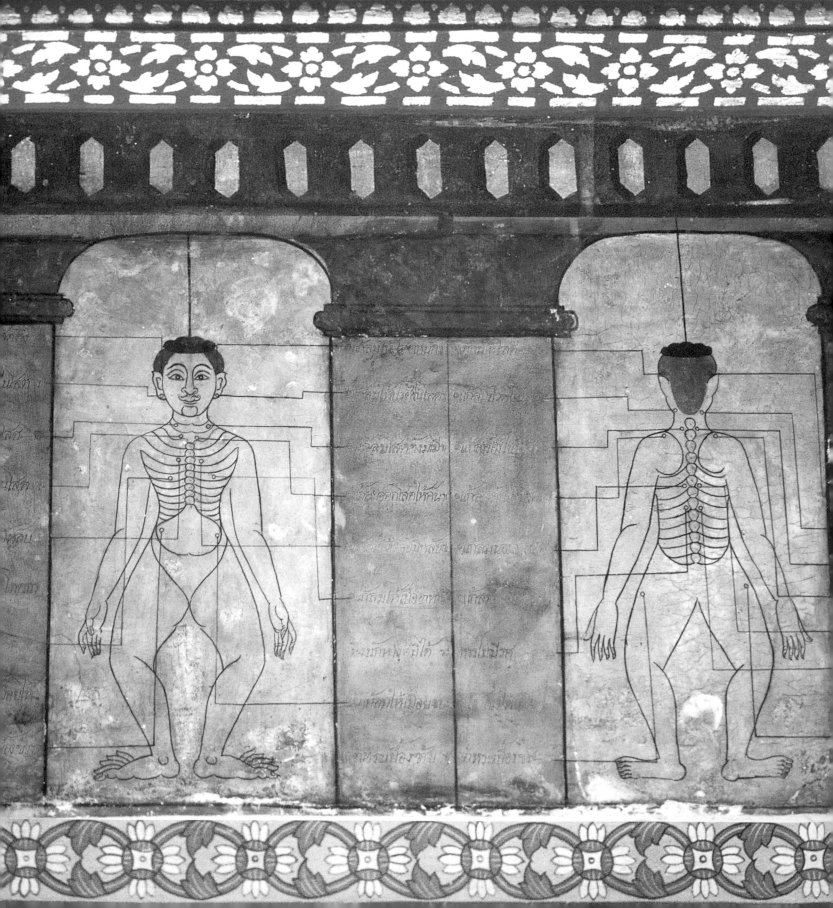

healing with the thai touch

Throughout rural Thailand, massage is a part of daily life. Massages are given with friendly abandon among family members and free massage sessions are available for the elderly at village temples. Thais treat a leisurely massage among kith and kin as a form of socialising that helps draw people together and strengthen the bonds within the community.

After all, it's a human instinct for people to touch and caress each other both for pleasure and to relieve pain and heal sickness. Thais have been practising this kind of natural massage in their communities for centuries.

What is known as Traditional Thai Massage is a formal healing art with roots in Theravada Buddhism, Thailand's national religion. The philosophy of traditional Thai massage originated as a spiritual practice derived from the teachings of Buddha, and in the early days was only taught and practised in temples. Even today, the most important massage school in Thailand is at Bangkok's Wat Po, or the Temple of the Reclining Buddha. Only recently have commercial massage schools begun operations.

When a masseur gives a Thai massage, he or she is practising the physical application of Metta, or 'loving kindness' advocated in Theravada Buddhism (see page 78). The masseur bestows his healing touch in the spirit of giving love. A truly good Thai masseur performs his art in a meditative mood, starting with a prayer to centre himself on the work he is about to perform. In this mood, he massages with meditative awareness, mindfulness and concentration. A massage performed thus differs vastly from other types of massage such as Swedish, sports, or aromatherapy, because it is this meditative mindfulness that gives the masseur the power to sense energy flows in the body and successfully treat the person according to his or her needs.

While it may appear that Thai massage requires great physical exertion from the masseur, when done properly, the giver isn't exhausted at all. Instead, the masseur is relaxed and refreshed, because Thai massage is an act of giving and compassion. By acting generously, a sense of well-being in generated — this nourishes both the giver and the recipient. When combined with a nutritious diet and healthy lifestyle, Thai massage may help a person reach (and maintain) a high level of fitness.

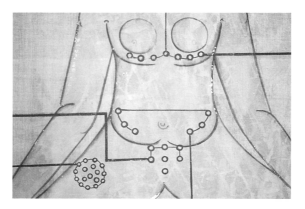

Left and opposite: Diagrams at Wat Po Massage School in Bangkok depict the energy lines and acupressure points along the body. During Thai massage, acupressure points are kneaded to release energy blockages.

an ancient healing art

Thai massage has its roots in ancient India, where it was practised over 2,500 years ago, well before the time of Buddha. It is believed that the founder of Thai massage was a doctor in northern India by the name of Shivaka Kumar Baccha who was the Buddha's personal medical advisor. His teachings on herbal medicine and massage arrived in Thailand along with Buddhist teachings by the first Buddhist monks and Brahmins around the 2nd or 3rd century BC.

Below: Statues at Wat Po Massage School depict various postures of the 'Hermit's Self Massage'. Derived from yoga poses, these postures show methods of self-massage that provide relief from a variety of ailments such as muscle cramps, tension and headache, waist pain, nausea, vertigo, and bodily discomforts caused by *wata*, or wind.

Once in Thailand, knowledge of this healing art spread and techniques were handed down orally from teacher to student. The ancient massage arts gradually gained a reputation for their abilities to alleviate backache, headache, stomach ache, and nervous tension, as well as more serious ailments such as fever, epileptic fits, early paralysis and speech defects.

Thai massage reached its peak about 200 years ago, then began to fall into a decline. It was revived by King Rama III (reigned 1824–1851) who had all existing knowledge about the techniques inscribed on stone tablets and erected at Wat Po in Bangkok, where they remain today. The tablets depict diagrams of the human body showing the body's key energy lines, where massage is applied to stimulate the circulation and effect healing. The practice began to flag again in the early 20th century, but was revived by King Rama VI (r 1910–1925), resulting in the establishment of two associations for traditional medicine and massage.

Technique-wise, Thai massage is based on the concept of invisible energy lines running along the body. This is linked to ancient Indian yoga philosophy, which states that we receive life energy, or *prana*, via a network of 72,000 energy lines that interconnect along our bodies. Thai massage focuses on ten key lines, known as *sip sen* (ten lines) in Thai.

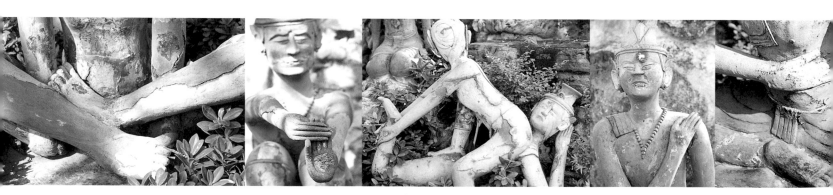

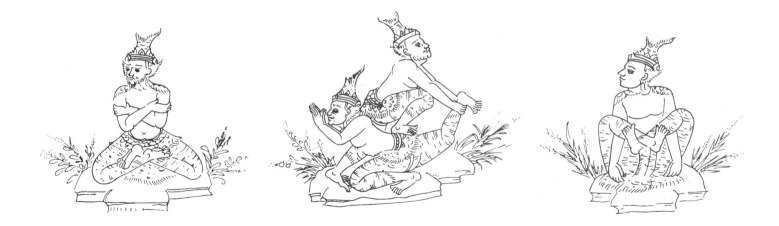

The energy along these lines powers all our physical, mental and emotional processes, so when there is an energy imbalance, the body's harmony is disrupted, causing pain and disease. Massaging along these energy lines can break energy blockages, stimulate the flow of *prana* and restore general well-being.

A key difference from western massage is that Thai massage is applied without oils, and the recipient remains fully clothed. Unlike the continuous strokes of western massage, the Thai method uses pressure, muscle stretching and compression, practised in gentle, rhythmic, rocking movements. All the movements are flowing and smooth. The masseur uses not just the hands, but also the feet, knees and elbows. The massage is usually performed on a mattress on the floor.

Some people complain of aching after a Thai massage in places where they didn't ache before. This is because when a person is suffering from internal stress or anxiety, muscle tension in the form of frowning, for example, may be so minute as to be unnoticeable. Prolonged tension results in headache, back ache or muscle pain in other parts of the body that become unnoticeable to the sufferer after a while. When these habitually tensed muscles are massaged, their energy blockages are released, thus resulting in discomfort. This can be remedied by a few more massage sessions.

There are six key aspects to traditional Thai massage, namely yoga, exercise, meditation, reflexology, acupressure and healing. The simple physical act of 'having a massage' is not the whole story. One needs to combine it with other physical, spiritual or mental activities — and then full benefits are attained.

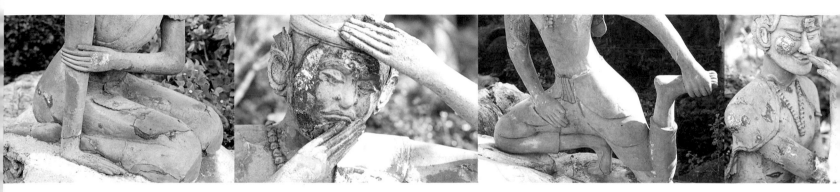

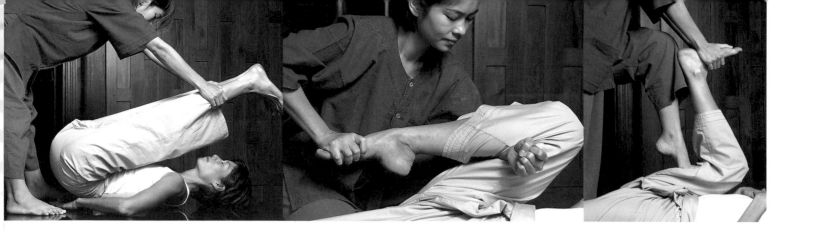

how to give a thai massage

"Giving a massage is a way of giving love through your hands," says Mae-Chee Sansanee, the founder of the Sathira-Dhammasthan Ashram in Bangkok. If you are keen to learn how to give a Thai massage, you will need to take a special course, but the most important starting point for the student is to first develop an empathy for other bodies. Each body differs from another and has unique needs.

Top: Thai massage is based on the stretching postures of yoga and doesn't make use of oil. The patient remains fully clothed in loose pyjamas to allow plenty of room for stretching. *Opposite:* Many leg-stretching postures elevate the legs while the body is lying on its back. This position alleviates low blood pressure and indigestion, and also stimulates the internal organs.

This is true in lots of cases. For instance, the yoga-like stretching performed in Thai massage may be pleasant for more flexible people, but could be harmful for those with stiff bodies. While some people may enjoy intense thumb pressure, others may find it painful. A focused masseuse needs to ask the receiver whether the pressure is comfortable or not, or whether it should be adjusted to a stronger or softer level.

For those who are interested in learning traditional techniques, there are two options. The first is a course at Wat Po Thai Traditional Medical School (Wat Po, Bangkok, tel: (66) 02-211-2974; email: watpottm@netscape.net); the second course we recommend is at The Foundation of

Shivago Komarpaj (Old Medical Hospital), near Chiang Mai Cultural Centre, Wualai Road, Chiang Mai; tel: (66) 053-235-085.

The Wat Po school offers three courses including general Thai massage, therapeutic and healing massage and foot massage. The first two types cover 30 hours of instruction and students can divide the duration into five-, six-, or ten-day courses. The foot massage course takes 15 hours and is taught within three days. In Chiang Mai, students can attend 12-day courses taught in English, which include a manual in English, and there are also long-term courses in the Thai language only, both in massage therapy and Ayurvedic medicine.

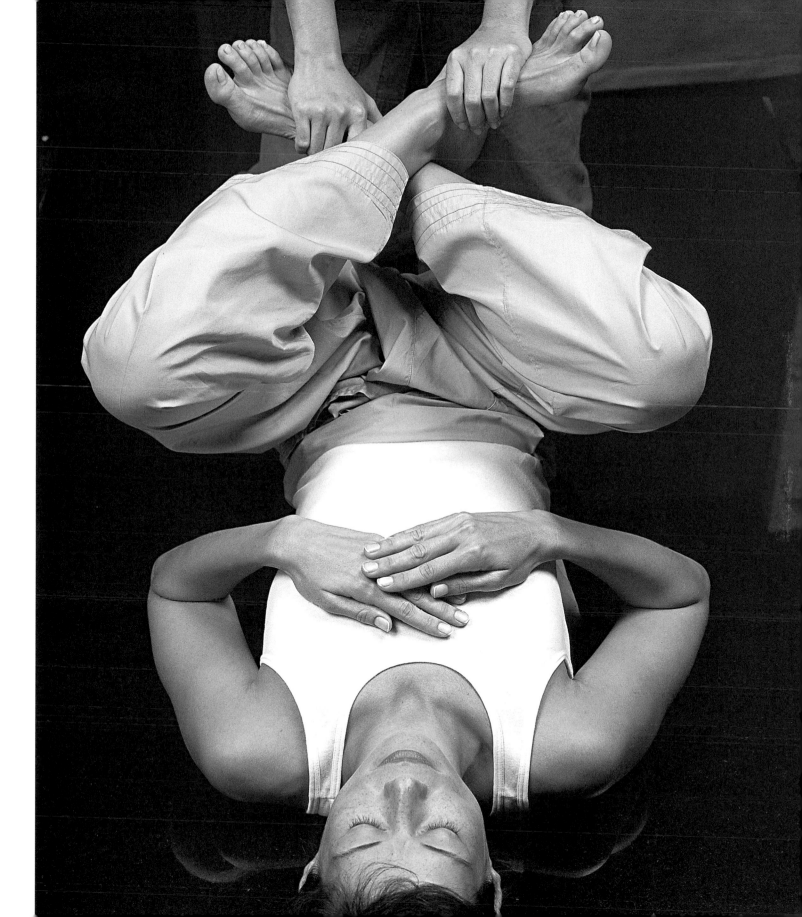

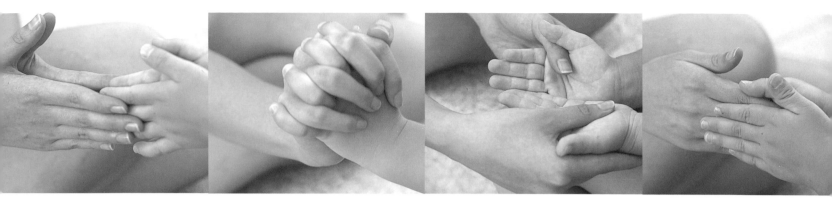

baby & child massage

A casual massage among family members at the end of the day has been a traditional way of relaxing in Thai households for centuries. In most families, it's customary for children to walk up and down the backs and legs of their parents and grandparents to massage their tired muscles. There is even an obscure custom of using cats to walk on their owners' backs, though the practice offers no real therapeutic benefits other than inducing a sense of relaxed fun.

As in most Asian cultures, babies and children are treated indulgently by Thai adults, and the pampering of children is as important in rearing a happy child as it is in developing the bond of filial devotion that is so intrinsic to Asian culture. Giving your child a massage can help lull a young one to sleep, soothe a troublesome tummy, and is a wonderful way of bonding between parent and child. It enhances the child's sense of well-being, and is often as soothing for the mother as it is for the child!

Babies love being hugged, kissed and stroked, and a massage is a natural extension of cuddling and playing with your baby. Babies have soft, silky skin that is a pleasure to touch. The easiest way to massage a baby's delicate little body is by using stroking movements with your hands, fingertips or thumbs. Keep your movements slow and smooth. There is no set sequence for a baby massage. Follow your instincts, and your baby's response should tell you what he or she enjoys.

The best oil to use on babies is a light vegetable oil such as sweet almond or sunflower oil. Baby oil is a mineral oil, and therefore not easily absorbed by the skin. An ideal time for a baby massage is after a bath, when he is relaxed and comfortable. He can lie in your lap or on a towel on the floor or bed.

Bliss for Baby

GENTLE LIMB MOVEMENTS
• Hold your baby's feet and bend and stretch each leg. Straighten the legs and gently push the knees together. Repeat a few times. Thais believe this prevents the development of bow-legs.
• Hold your baby's hands and cross his arms over his chest. Take the arms out to the sides and stretch them. Bring the arms up in the air, then cross them again. Bring the arms above the head and stretch.

ARMS AND LEGS
• Hold up one arm and stroke from the shoulder to the hand, then squeeze gently all over. Stroke the back of the hand, then uncurl the fingers and gently squeeze and rotate each finger.
• Lift one leg and stroke and squeeze it all over. Stroke the foot, then squeeze and rotate each toe.

FACE
• Stroke the baby's forehead from the centre to the sides. Then stroke from the nose, out to the temples; glide down the sides to the chin.
• Circle around the eyes, stroking out along the eyebrows and very gently back under the eyes. Then press gently on the temples.

BACK
• Lie your baby on his tummy and stroke the whole back, starting from the feet and stroking up to the shoulders and down the arms. Then glide your hands gently down the sides.
• Glide your hands gently across the back in a criss-crossing movement. Glide your hands smoothly down the back, one hand after the other. As one hand reaches the legs, lift it, return to the neck and repeat.

ABDOMEN
• Stroke from the thighs up the front of the body, glide your hands out to the shoulders, down the arms, then down the sides of the body.

• Place both hands on either side of the body with fingers pointing toward each other. Glide your hands lightly back and forth across the abdomen in a criss-crossing movement.
• Stroke clockwise in a circle around the navel with one hand after the other. This soothing movement is good for relieving upset stomachs.

Time for the Children
Children enjoy being massaged too, as it makes them feel pampered and loved. There are no set rules for massaging children, as long as the child enjoys it. A good time to give your child a massage is at bedtime, and you can give the massage while the child is wearing pyjamas.

ABDOMEN
• Gently stroke the tummy, gliding your hands up the chest. Massaging your child in smooth, clockwise strokes around the navel can help soothe a stomach ache. Always stroke clockwise around the stomach, as this is the direction food moves through the digestive system, but never do this right after a meal.

BACK
• Stroke up the back and glide down the sides of your child's body. Gently knead the shoulders, then stroke out over the tops of the arms. Repeat.

LEGS AND FEET
• Stroke and squeeze down the legs and then massage the feet. With the child on his tummy and knees bent so that the soles of the feet face the ceiling, gently chop down on the soles of the feet with the sides of your hand.

HANDS
• Massage the hands by squeezing and rotating each finger, then stroking the palm.

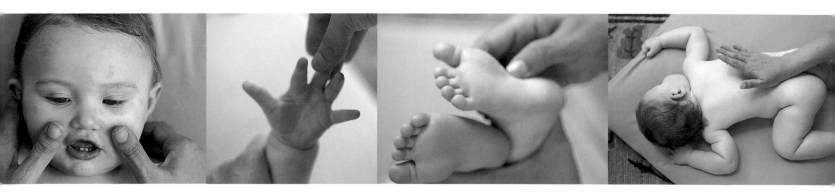

reflexology

Foot massage is so popular in Thailand that it seems you can find a foot massage establishment on just about any street corner in any Thai city. While at some you may get at best a relaxing foot massage, at others you may find dedicated, professional reflexology. Most of the major spas in Thailand offer reflexology massage for the feet, a healing massage that can leave not just your feet, but your whole body walking on air.

Reflexology is a holistic therapy that applies pressure to specific points of the feet to treat problems in all parts of the body. Similar to the concept of Thai massage therapy, reflexology is based on the principle that the body has natural energy that flows freely around the body when the person is in good health. The body's energy flows in zones and is dynamic, balancing itself to meet the individual's needs. With stress, tension, anxiety,

poor diet, or lack of exercise, the energy flow becomes disrupted. In reflexology, specific points on the feet and hands are thought to correspond to each part of the body. Applying pressure to points on the foot is supposed to treat the corresponding part of the body.

Though the practice of foot massage has been known to man since the earliest civilizations and is depicted on Egyptian tomb paintings, reflexology as

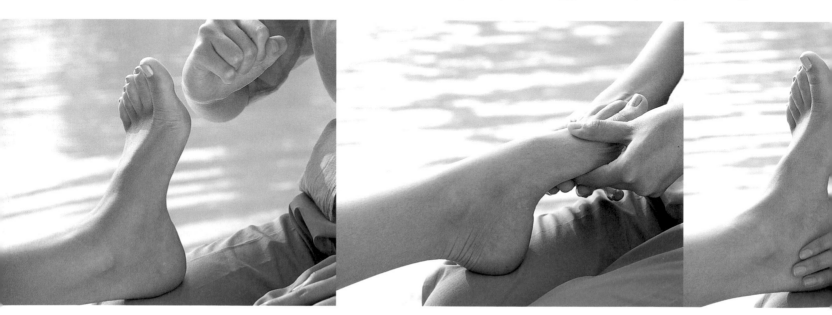

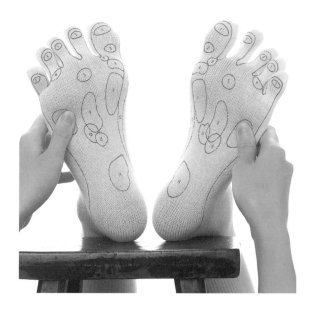

we know it today is a modern therapy developed in the early 20th century. It was an American woman, Eunice Ingham, who identified and mapped out the body's reflex zones in a form of zone therapy, referring to the method as reflexology.

How can a reflexologist tell when there's an energy block in your body? One sign of energy imbalance is a gritty feeling, crystal-like in texture, that the reflexologist can detect beneath the skin. The location of the grittiness indicates the problem area in the body. The reflexologist will try to break down this grittiness in order to restore the energy flow to that part of the body and flush out the toxins. The patient may feel discomfort when pressure is applied to problem spots. This helps the therapist identify the origin of the imbalance in the body, and treat that area by releasing the energy block there.

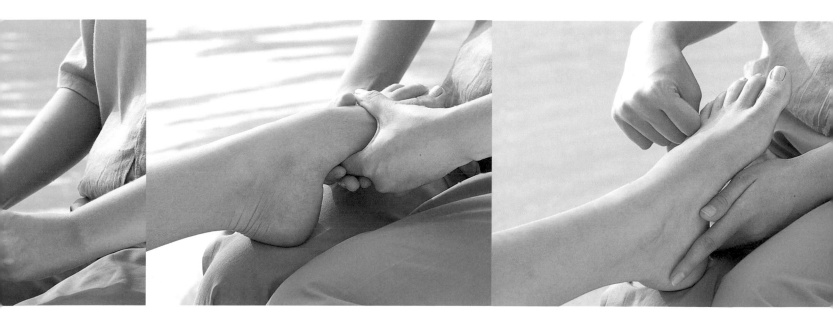

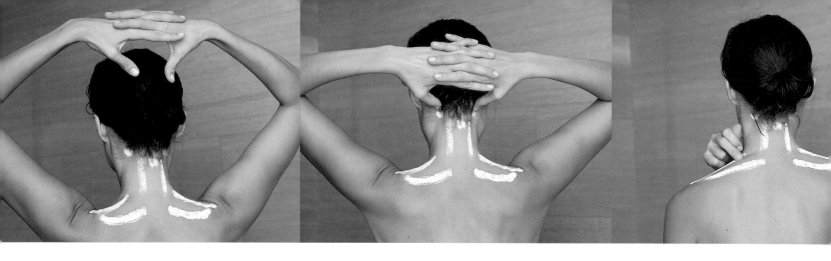

do-it-yourself massage

At The Banyan Tree Phuket, guests at the luxurious new spa pool villas enjoy the privacy of a swimming pool and spa treatments in their own outdoor massage pavilions. Among the special services provided to guests staying at the spa pool villas is a half-hour massage lesson, based on the principles of traditional Thai massage, and taught by professional massage instructors from the Banyan Tree Spa Academy. Sharing a massage lesson and practising with your partner or friend is a wonderful bonding experience. But you don't always need another person to get a relaxing massage — for a quick pick-me-up, it's quite simple and very effective to give yourself a massage! The Banyan Tree Spa Academy offers the following tips for self-massage techniques that can be easily done while sitting at your desk or relaxing at home. The following techniques work on the acupressure points on the neck, shoulders, face and head.

TENSION RELIEF MASSAGE FOR THE NECK

This Neck Tension Relief Massage works on the pressure points at the base of your skull and helps relieve headaches and tension in the neck.

1. Lock the fingers of both hands together, leaving both thumbs free. Place the locked hands behind your head.
2. Keeping your head straight, start by pressing the pressure points at the base of your hairline between your ears and your spine. Press both thumbs very slowly, in small, circular motions for 10 seconds and end by pushing both thumbs upward in a swift, brushing movement.

3. Move your thumbs about an inch inwards towards the spine and slowly repeat this motion.
4. When you reach the spine, place each thumb on either side of the spine and slowly repeat this motion down along both sides of the spine.
5. Repeat this motion downward and then upwards again.
6. After a while you should start to feel relaxed. End the massage when both thumbs reach the base of the hairline at the top of the spine. You will find a natural depression at the top of the spine, directly below the base of the skull. Press both thumbs into the depression, and quickly brush thumbs upwards 3 to 4 times, to release energy there.

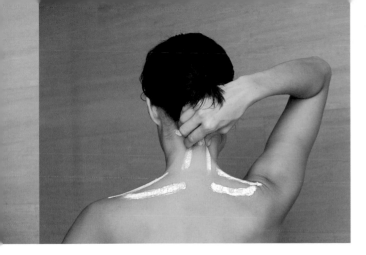

SHOULDER MASSAGE

This Shoulder Massage relieves tension on the back of your shoulders. It works on the energy lines running along the top of your shoulders and down your shoulder blades, where muscle knots can form from long hours of sitting at a desk or at the computer.

1. Cross your right arm across your chest and reach your right hand over your left shoulder.
2. Use your right middle finger to locate any tension knots along the area between the shoulder blade and spine.
3. Press your finger firmly in slow, circular motions around this area, working on knotted muscles.
4. Repeat the same motions on the other side, with your left arm crossing your chest to work on your right shoulder.

FACE MASSAGE

This Face Massage helps relieve the tension of frowning that occurs when you have been concentrating too hard on your work or while reading. The massage works on the acupressure points along your brow bone.

1. Interlock the fingers of both hands, leaving your thumbs free. With elbows pointed outward and towards your sides, place each thumb on the inside of the brow bone on each eye. Press in firmly.
2. Slowly and firmly slide your thumbs in one motion along the brow bone of each eye until you reach your temples on either side of your head.
3. Press thumbs into each temple in small, firm, circular motions for a minute or two, or until you feel some relief from tension.
4. Slowly repeat this motion with both thumbs moving toward the back of your head, until both thumbs reach the centre of the back of the head.
5. Keep repeating this massage, starting from your inside brow bone, until you feel better.

HEAD AND SCALP MASSAGE

The Head and Scalp Massage is a highly relaxing massage that is given at the end of every traditional Thai massage session. It helps relieve headaches and stimulates the nerves in the head. It exercises the scalp, stimulating the blood circulation in the head to promote hair growth. It also strengthens the roots of the hair and is thought to help prevent baldness.

1. Starting at the temples, grab a handful of hair on each side of the head, about an inch from the scalp. Slowly pull along the hair, gradually adding pressure as you move your hands along the length of the hair away from the scalp.
2. Repeat this motion on both sides of your head, continually moving backwards until you reach the centre of the back of your head.
3. Starting from the hairline on your forehead, repeat this motion along the top of your head, moving backwards all the time.

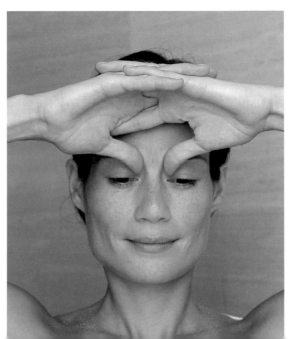

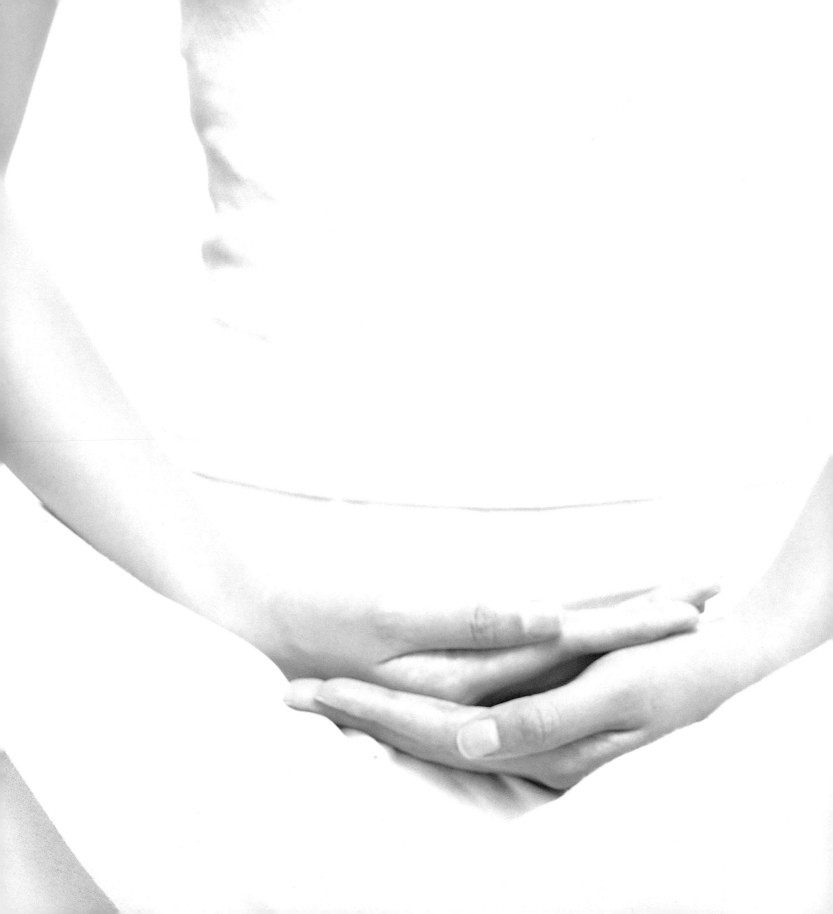

the path to serenity

"The power of the mind comes from pure, still focus — not simply from the gesture of a hand or a sitting pose. Your power comes from the inner being."
— *Mae Chee Sansanee, Buddhist nun and founder of Sathira-Dhammasthan Ashram*

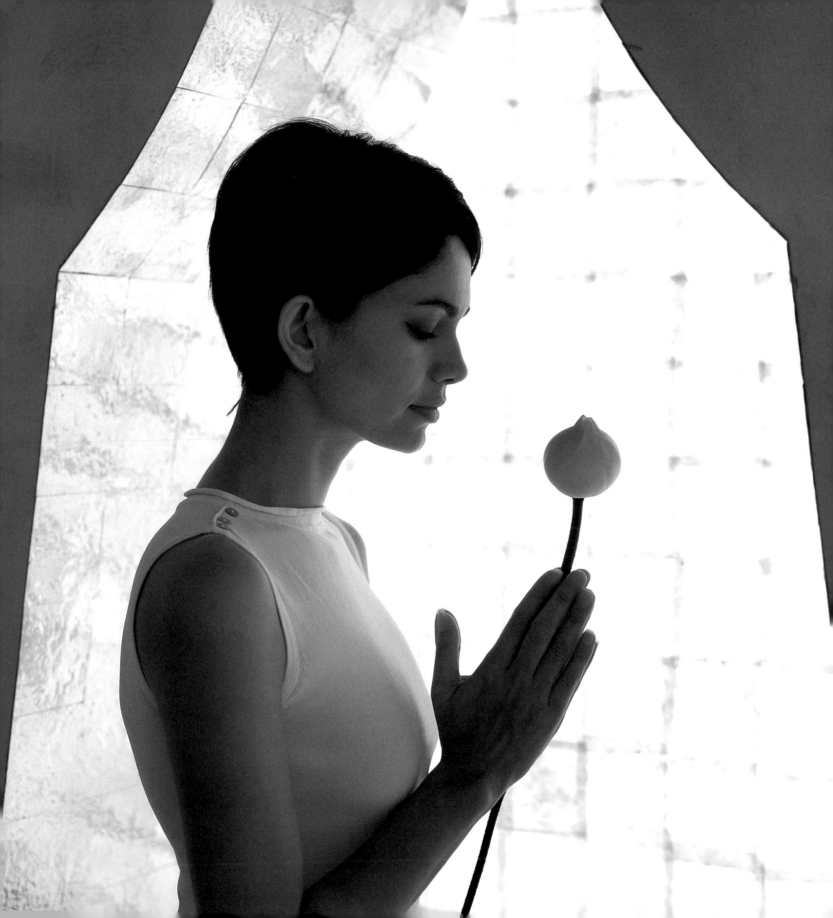

mind, body & spirit

The sights and symbols of Thai culture are laden with images of a rich spirituality. Thais are predominantly Buddhist and practice their faith as a way of life. But though the image of meditation is most often linked to the Buddhist religion, meditation itself does not require Buddhist faith or belief. Meditation is a path, not a goal in itself. It doesn't necessarily mean sitting cross-legged chanting a mantra, though that's the image most associated with the practice.

Meditation is the path through which the Buddhist faith developed. Buddhism evolved from the meditations of Siddhartha Gautama, an Indian prince who rejected the material world, and through meditation experienced a transformation that brought him to enlightenment, or Buddha-hood, around the fifth century BC. Meditation remains central to most, though by no means all, Buddhist practices.

In the Thai Buddhist tradition, Buddha is regarded as an earthly being and a teacher, not a deity. The word Buddha means 'awakened', and refers not to the person, but to the state of enlightenment of the awakened one and the awakened state. This means there's a Buddha mind within us all. It's not something we have to create — it's already there, and meditation helps give us access to the potential Buddha within us. In the Buddhist tradition, meditation is a path to reach a state of enlightenment, but even if you don't aspire to reach such heights, the practice of meditation can have a calming influence in your daily life.

The Buddha identified over a hundred types of meditation, of which approximately 40 are considered the main practices in the Theravada tradition, which is the school of Buddhism practised in Thailand. While there are many schools and styles of meditation, the forms of meditation most familiar to Thais are those that are central to Buddhism. In the following pages we explain some of the tenets and practices.

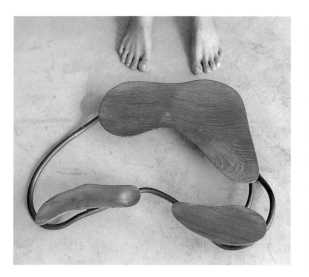

Opposite: The lotus is the sacred flower for both Buddhists and Hindus. It symbolises purity and is presented to Buddha figures as a religious offering in Thailand.
Left: Designed specifically for meditation, this chair is a sculpture. Its design supports the body in the lotus position when seated in the chair, and is one of a pair now belonging in a private collection in Bangkok.

buddhist meditation

In the Theravada Buddhism tradition, the various meditative practices can be grouped into two main types. Samatha or Tranquility Meditation, and Vipassana or Insight Meditation. The first type calms the mind, the second allows one to free oneself from the mind.

Samatha (Tranquility Meditation)

In this form of meditation, a state of calming the mind is reached by training your attention to fixate on an object. The focus of attention can be on something in the present moment, such as a flower, a candle, a sound or your own breath. Through the practice of mindful focus, the restless mind is calmed.

During our every day life, our senses are bombarded with external stimuli and our thoughts are constantly active, often thinking several different thoughts at the same time. We are conditioned by our thoughts, most of the time remaining unaware of how they imprison us. The practice of Tranquility Meditation helps us still the mind, letting us experience its calm state. This allows us to become aware of how thoughts and impulses are generated though our minds. Thus as we meditate, our thoughts become more clear and calm and our ability to focus improves. During periods of stress, unhappiness or confusion, this type of meditation helps bring about a sense of calm, inner peace and awareness.

Practioners of Tranquility Meditation note that their ability to focus improves, as does their mental clarity and peace of mind. Because they can concentrate better, anxiety is alleviated and depression may be eased.

Vipassana (Insight Meditation)

There are various schools of Buddhism, but at their core is the teaching of Vipassana, the representative meditation practice of the Theravada school of Buddhism. In Pali, the ancient language used in the Theravada Buddhist scriptures, the word *vipassana* means 'insight'. It is a practical method for developing self knowledge through a form of self-observation known as mindfulness.

Vipassana is also called Insight Meditation. The first step is to develop steadiness of mind with the preliminary practice of Samatha Meditation. Then one can move on to Tranquility Meditation — clearing up mental clutter, focusing and allowing one to move on to Insight Meditation, which opens up the mind's awareness. Vipassana helps one to observe the calmed mind, to understand its nature and to achieve awareness of its workings and processes. Mindful awareness is the goal of all Buddhist practice, and the key to enlightenment.

In Insight Meditation, the calm mind becomes aware of the thoughts and impulses generated by it, thus providing the insight to free oneself from the shackles of the mind. Practioners report greater self-awareness, mindful attention in everyday life, an insight into the nature of the mind, as well as the ability to recognise negative habits of the mind.

Opposite: The lotus position is usually done while seated on the ground, as shown here in the serene atmosphere of the lobby of the Devarana Spa, Bangkok.

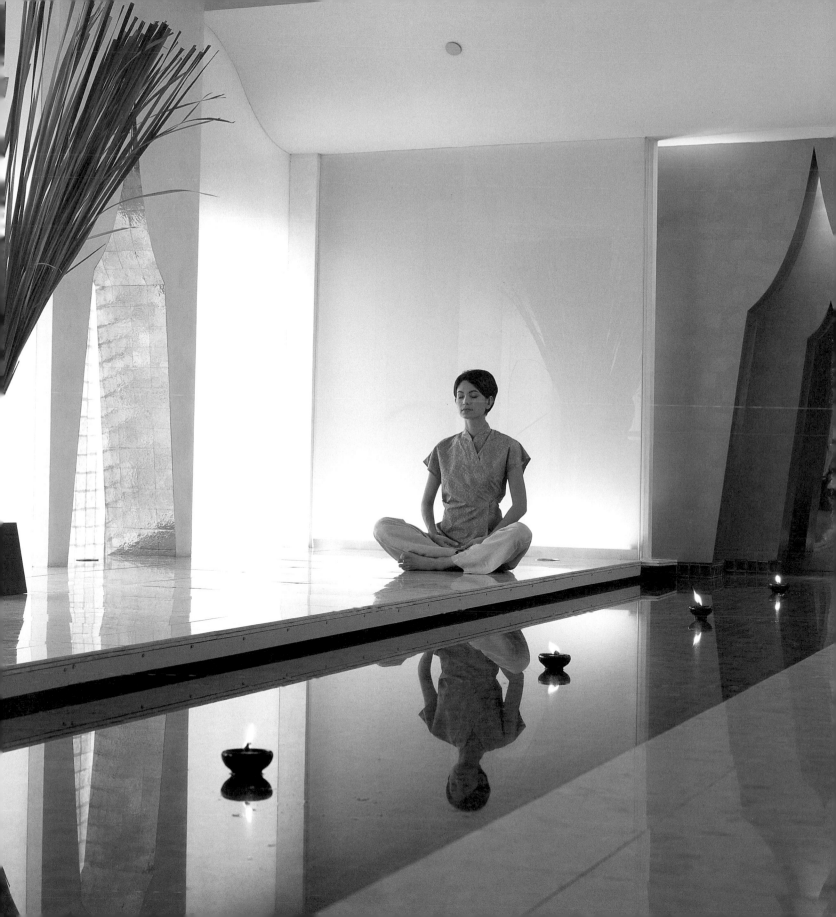

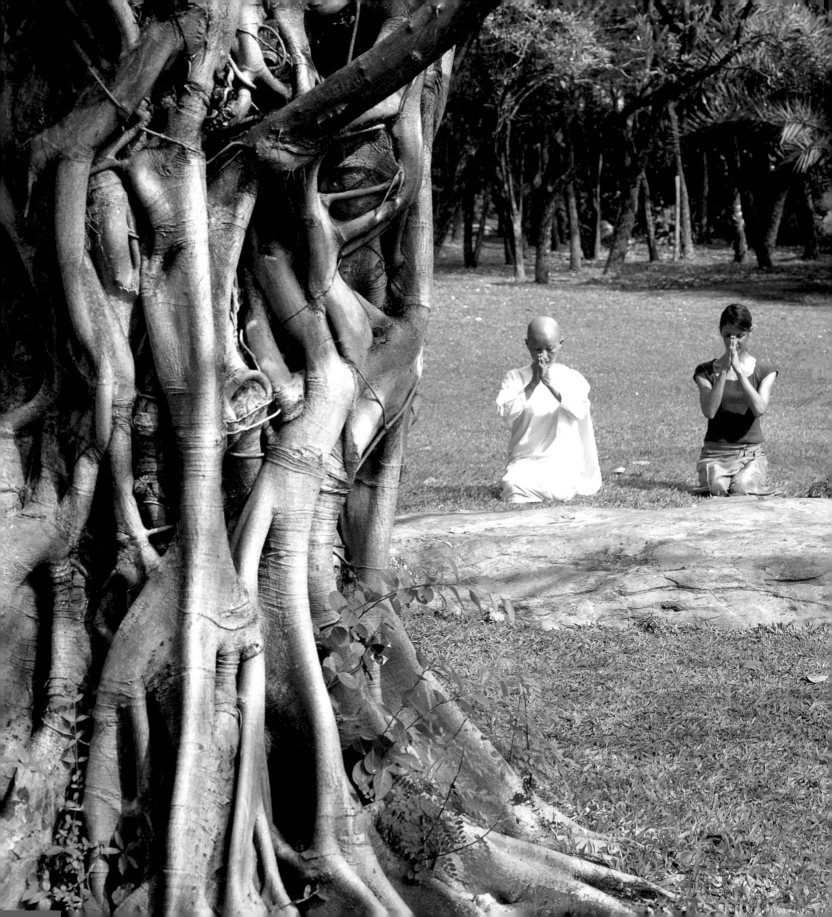

Vipassana is also known as Mindfulness Meditation, though they aren't exactly one and the same. The practice of mindfulness is part of the greater technique of Vipassana, and most schools of Buddhism consider mindfulness to be the foundation of Vipassana. Mindfulness is the practice that leads to greater awareness of thoughts and emotions, thus enabling one to recognise the thought conditioning of daily life. During the process of mindfulness, awareness is focused on mindful attention and observation of the present moment, the here and now. Thus, the mind attains a greater freedom from its thoughts and disturbing emotions, and its natural wisdom is free to emerge.

In our everyday life, we tend to cling to habits, labels, obsessions, addictions and compulsions. We cling to what we perceive to be emotional and mental security, perhaps even to dysfunctional relationships or jobs. Mindfulness allows us to drop our pre-conditioned habits of the mind. It allows us to experience a shift in consciousness and glimpse the reality of who and what we are. Thus,

mindfulness liberates us by restoring us to the spacious quality of the mind.

There are four foundations of mindfulness contemplation: body, feeling, mind and mental phenomena. They are known as the Satipatthana, or 'foundation of mindfulness', because we generate experiences from these four components, even though we may not be aware of them. For example, when eating lunch, one's mind is busy processing other thoughts, unaware of the actual here and now experience of what is going on in the body, mind, feelings and mental phenomena. By focusing on and observing the process of these four objects, mindfulness can be developed.

Mindfulness of breathing is one way to practice these four foundations. Here, we focus on the breath. By observing the breath, we become aware of the experience of our body as we breathe, our feeling of breathing, our mind and our mental state.

When you start focusing your mind on a meditation object such as your breath, it allows you to see how restless the mind is, because in the

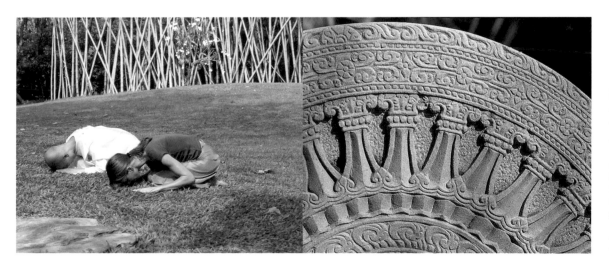

Opposite and far left: The Buddha attained enlightenment meditating underneath a Bodhi tree, such as the one shown here at the Sathira Dhammasthan Ashram, Bangkok. The Bodhi is therefore a sacred tree for Buddhists. *Left:* An important motif in Buddhist art, the wheel symbolises the Buddha's enlightenment; his first sermon was called "Setting in Motion the Wheel of the Truth".

attempt to focus on one object, you become aware of how the mind keeps jumping from one thought to another. The point is to become aware of the restlessness, and the restlessness will eventually subside. The breath is very important because it sustains life to the body. Therefore, in meditative practice, mastering the breath is an indirect way of mastering the mind. Regulating the flow of breath through mindfulness breathing makes the breath calm, thus relaxing the mind. Mindfulness of breathing incorporates both Tranquility and Insight Meditation practices; you anchor your mind on your breath, while using it as a basis to generate mindfulness towards all four foundations.

Tips on Mindfulness Practice:
• practice at the same time every day
• choose a peaceful, quiet place to practice
• sit comfortably, but erect, with eyes closed

• pay attention to your body and any sensations
• pay attention to your breath
• pay attention to the sounds you hear
• direct your attention to the contents of your mind, and observe any thoughts that may arise
• when your mind wanders, gently return to the practice with a sense of forgiveness and compassion to yourself. Do not berate yourself for losing focus.

Metta (Loving Kindness Meditation)

Most Thais, as Buddhists, are familiar with the word Metta, or 'loving kindness'. To Thais this is a beautiful word, also given as a name to girls. The Buddhist faith preaches the value of loving others, and there is a form of Buddhist meditation practice called Metta Meditation. While the conventional idea of love tends to connote possessiveness of the

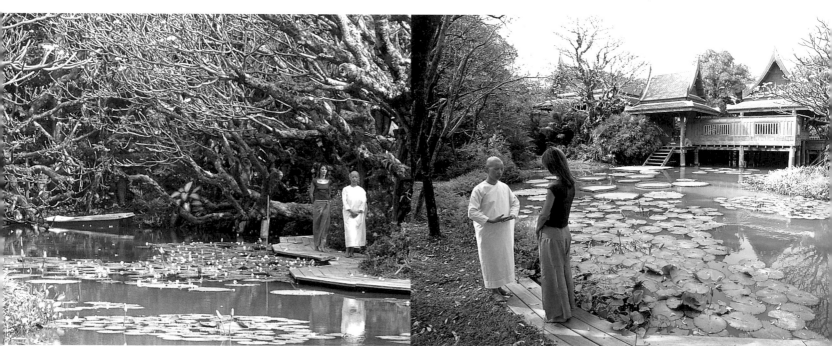

being or object that is loved, Metta is different in that it embraces all beings. Metta is more like a spiritual love that helps you see the good in others, having loving kindness for others as sentient beings.

Metta begins with learning how to love yourself, by awakening loving kindness within yourself, toward yourself. This helps you feel strong enough to expand your loving kindness towards others. The practice of Metta brings serenity and good will to your consciousness. It makes other people friendlier toward you, and helps make you less judgmental towards yourself and others. Metta is a form of spiritual healing, because the cultivation of loving kindness is a remedy for fear. Instead of just trying to heal yourself, you're trying to heal others too.

The practice of Metta meditation also makes a good start from which to begin your journey through the different levels of meditation practice.

When you begin your meditation experience with the self-forgiveness that comes with Metta practice, you experience a calmness that comes with a sense of being at peace with yourself and the world around you. Thus it becomes easier for your mind to move into the focused state that is required of Tranquility and Insight Meditation practices.

Tips on Loving Kindness Meditation:
• begin by comforting yourself to be strong enough to expand your loving kindness towards others.
• when you direct loving kindness toward others, it's important to realize that all human beings have the same flesh and blood, and a desire for happiness.
• When you realise that other beings experience life with the same feelings as you do, you begin to appreciate the feeling of connectedness, and you feel that harming others is the same as harming yourself. That is the perspective of loving kindness.

Below. The tranquil gardens of Sathira Dhammasthan Ashram in Bangkok provide a peaceful place for the community. The garden includes a series of 'mindful steps' — uneven steps that help draw the walker's attention to each step, thus using the ordinary act of walking as an object of meditation training.

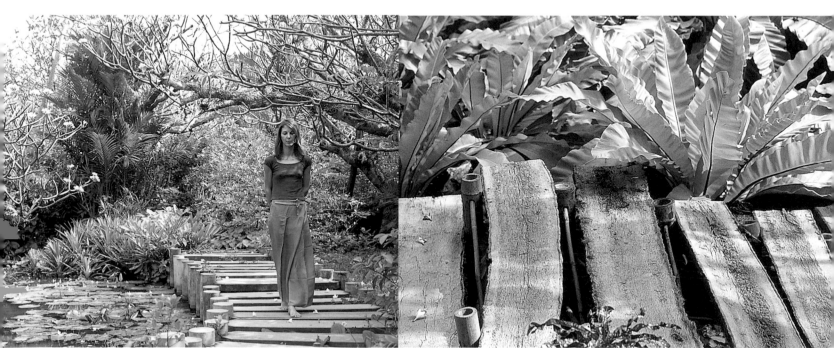

centre of concentration

For those who want to delve deeper into the mind-body-spirit conundrum, Thailand offers opportunities for exploration. We give you some ideas of exactly what is — and isn't — possible.

The Sathira-Dhammasthan Ashram in Bangkok is a community spiritual centre founded by the Buddhist nun Mae-Chee Sansanee, a former well-known actress and television personality who left the secular world to follow a spiritual life. Located in seven acres of tranquil gardens in the midst of Bangkok, the ashram has become a centre for the community to learn and practice living in harmony and compassion. It is a community where the concept and practice of Dhamma provides the focus and driving force for spiritual development.

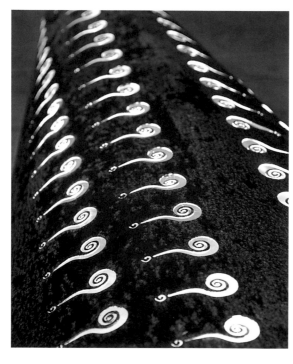

Right and opposite: These two works are part of a signature series by renowned Thai artist Montien Boonma. 'Black Question' (right) focuses on question marks, thus calling on the audience to examine their beliefs. "Sala of the Mind" (opposite) was inspired by the Khmer *prangs* at Angkor Wat, and provides a space for the audience to rest their mind and thoughts, thus allowing them to be in a *sala*, or room of the mind.

The ashram has three main programmes consisting of nine activities, covering all ages and genders. Each of the programmes is based on the principles of caring, sharing and respect.

1. A Beautiful World Begins with Dhamma — an ongoing retreat in the art of living through meditation and the teaching of Dhamma. This programme strengthens participants' well-being, security and serenity to form a solid base for inner peace.

2. Building a Better World Through Children — a programme that centres on children and parents, extended families, and communities together to participate in daily life activities. Underprivileged and special-needs children are involved in these projects, not only as recipients but also as an inspiration and humbling example to those more fortunate than they.

3. A Beautiful World Begins With Compassionate Service — a programme that develops volunteers and offers them an opportunity to gain fulfilment through service to others as a path to inner peace.

Sathira-Dhammasthan Ashram,
24/5 Soi Wacharaphon, Ramindra 55 Road,
Bangkok 10230, Thailand.
Tel: (66) 02 510-6697, 02 510-4756, 02 509-2237
Fax: (66) 02 519-4633
Email: savika@loxinfo.co.th

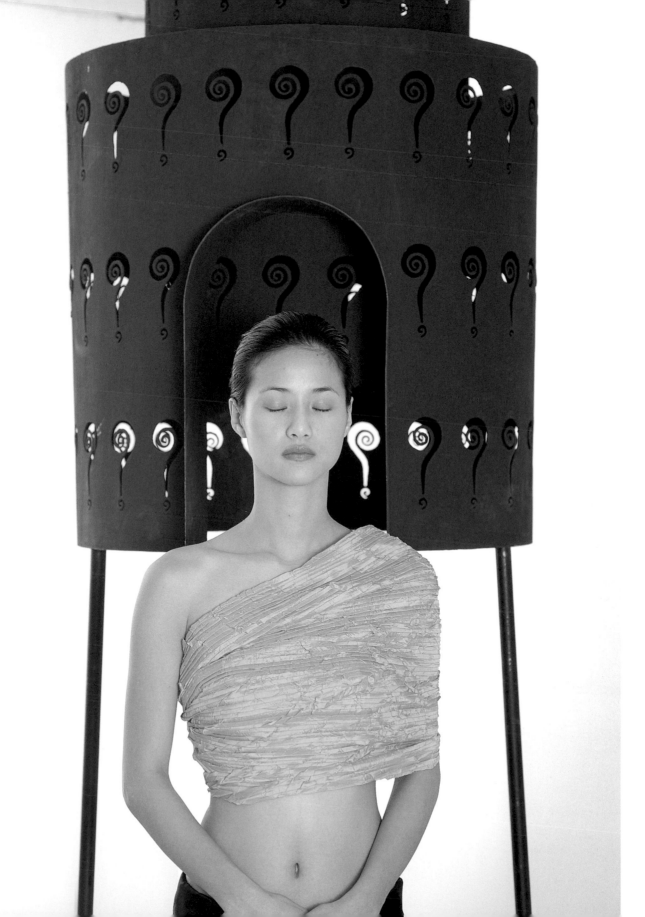

yoga

Today no self-respecting spa would be complete without courses in yoga as part of its mind-body therapies. Although not a Thai traditional therapy, it has a vital presence in Thai spas. So, what exactly is yoga?

Yoga is a system of spiritual, mental and physical practice that is a holistic approach to well-being. More than just a set of contortions for the body, it is a lifestyle, a way of thinking, and a way of being with the world. Yoga's purpose is to strengthen the body and make it more flexible, as well as awaken the spirit.

With its roots in India, some of the concepts of this ancient Indian yoga philosophy were brought to Thailand along with the healing traditions accompanying the influx of Buddhism in the 2nd and 3rd centuries BC. That is why Thai traditional massage incorporates a number of yoga stretching poses to improve flexibility to the muscles and spine.

The word 'yoga' is derived from the Sanskrit for 'union', and yoga has as its aim the realisation of oneness with the universe. Yoga originated in India over 5,000 years ago and played an integral part in the growth of Hinduism, Buddhism and the Indian civilisation as a whole. It is a system of

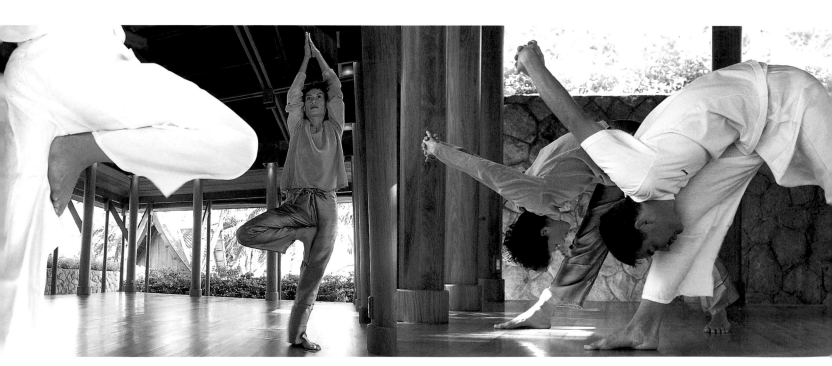

physical poses (*asanas*), breathing techniques (*pranayama*) and meditation. When the exercises and postures are practised regularly, it tones the muscles and improves posture, movement and balance. The entire process brings with it healing effects on the body and mind.

An important aspect of yoga is the belief in the *prana*, or 'life force', which is believed to be the universal energy that flows through everything, giving life and form to matter and spirit. According to yoga practioners, we participate in the flow of *prana* when we breathe, hence the breathing system plays an important part in the practice of yoga. Yoga breathing exercises, or *pranayama*, are fundamental to inner harmony and health. They are designed to direct the flow of *prana* and to release the body's internal energy to create spiritual awareness. The poses, meditation and breathing are only a small part of the overall philosophy and practice of yoga.

Below: The standing *asanas*, or yoga poses, stretch and strengthen the back, shoulders, and leg muscles. They improve posture, balance and muscular coordination, and are particularly useful for those with back stiffness or people who spend too much time sitting down.

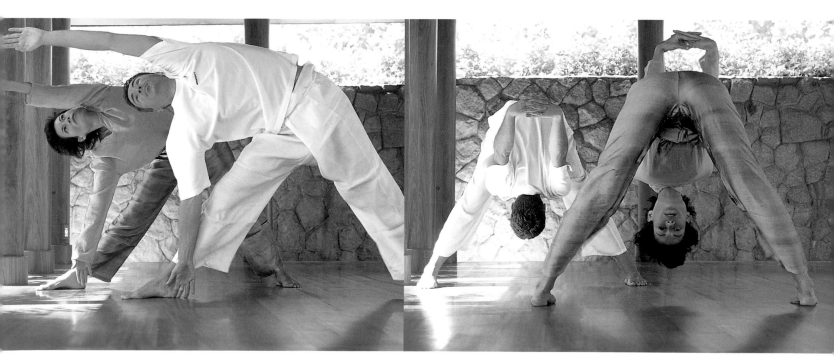

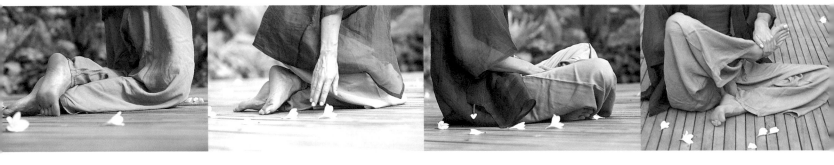

Yoga Asanas

Hatha yoga is a practice in which the physical body is used to achieve greater awareness by assuming postures, called *asanas*, and becoming aware of their sensations. The physical demands of the *asanas* give your body physical fitness, but more than that, they create a balance in the energy of the body and mind. Yoga training gives you strength and flexibility that comes from an inner vitality that gives you flowing energy. The practice of Hatha yoga prepares the body for the physical discipline of long periods of sitting meditation practice.

Yoga Breathing, or *Pranayama*

Pranayama is a Sanskrit word that means the control of the breath. The Yoga Sutras say that the disturbances of the mind cause irregular breathing, while regular breathing leads to tranquility, thus preparing the mind for meditation. The lungs are one of the organs of the excretory system; they remove waste products like carbon dioxide from

the body. Breathing deeply not only calms the mind, it helps prevent disease on a physical level, thus breathing is a form of self-healing for the mind and body.

During *pranayama* breathing, the movement of your breath massages your whole body. Many of us don't breathe properly because our breathing is blocked by inhibitions or tension. When you are tense or stressed, the capillaries in the body become blocked and blood flow is constricted due to the hard, tight, rigid muscles that result from the tension. When breathing is relaxed, it enhances the flow of blood and oxygen in your body, thus giving you more energy and leading to life force.

Benefits of Yoga

Yoga is not a therapy for specific illnesses, but the practice can bring about general improvements to your body functioning and well being. Practitioners report both mental and physical benefits, but stress that yoga needs to become part of one's

Above: When going from a standing position to a sitting position during meditation, the movements should be slow and fluid. The ideal position for sitting meditation is the full lotus position — sitting cross-legged with each foot on the opposite thigh, soles facing up. This position gives the best balance for the body and is most suitable for long periods of sitting.

"Most people suffer from wrong thinking and wrong goals in life. Happiness doesn't come from external possessions...when you have peace of mind, your beauty will radiate from within."
— *Mae Chee Sansanee, Buddhist nun and founder of Sathira-Dhammasthan Ashram*

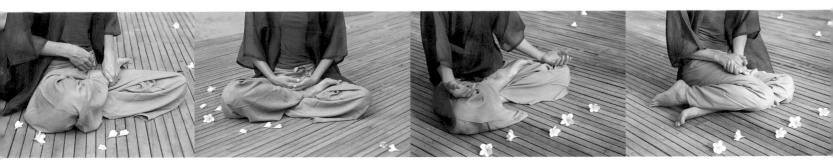

way of life. It cannot be practised irregularly. Physiological benefits include:

- Stabilisation of the nervous system
- Decrease in pulse rate, respiratory rate, blood pressure
- Cardiovascular and respiratory efficiency increases
- Balancing of the endocrine and digestive systems
- Normalization of weight
- Increase of muscular flexibility and joint movement
- Improvement of posture, better sleep
- Increase in energy, strength, endurance and immunity

Psychological benefits include:

- Decrease in anxiety, depression and hostility
- Improvement in mood and general sense of well-being
- Improvement in attention span, concentration, memory

Yoga's Anti-Aging Benefits

According to yoga philosophy, it's the flexibility of the spine, not the number of years, that determines a person's age. Yoga retards the aging process by giving elasticity to the spine, firming up the skin, removing tension from the body, strengthening the abdominal muscles, improving muscle tone, and poor posture — all the characteristics of youth!

It has been proven scientifically that yoga has a rejuvenating effect on the pituitary, thyroid, adrenal, sex glands and nervous system. When the functioning of these glands improve, your body realises a sense of well-being, and you attain a more positive mental and emotional state. This helps you feel more confident, relaxed, and optimistic in your everyday life. The proper practice of yoga can uplift your spirit — small wonder that the Madonnas and Mariahs of this world are devotees!

Above far right: Between postures, one should take up the correct sitting position — legs at the side, and hands clasped together at rest on the right leg.

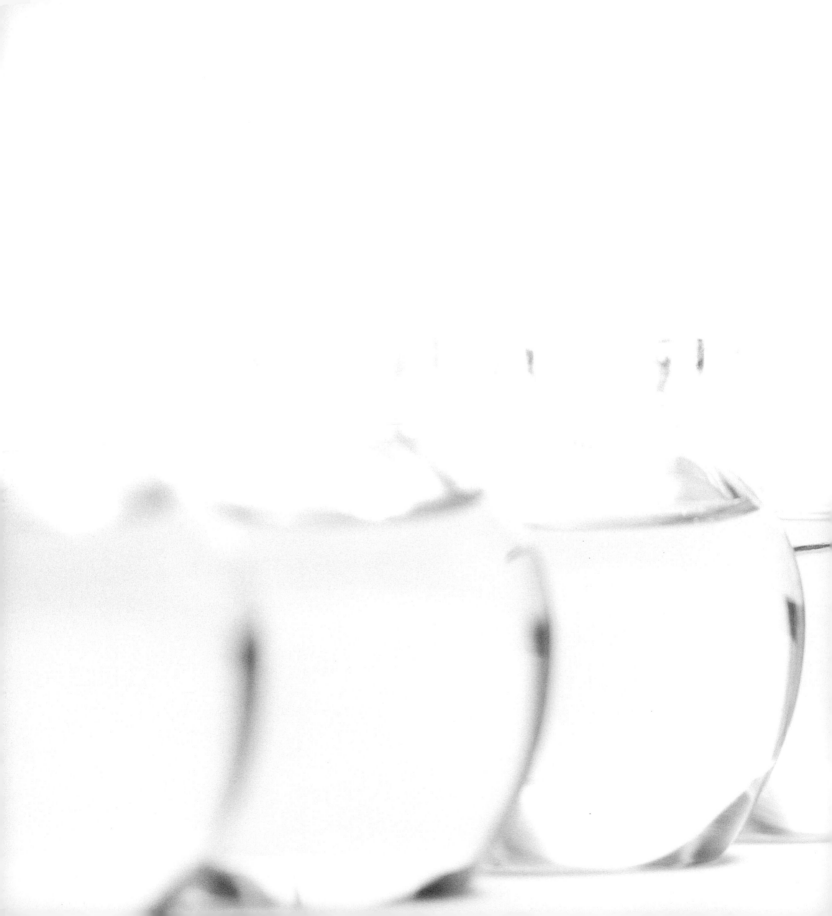

the thai spa at home

"Daily care of your own body is the best pampering of all — be good to yourself, because you deserve it."
— *Khun Orawan Choeysawat, spa manager, The Oriental Spa,*

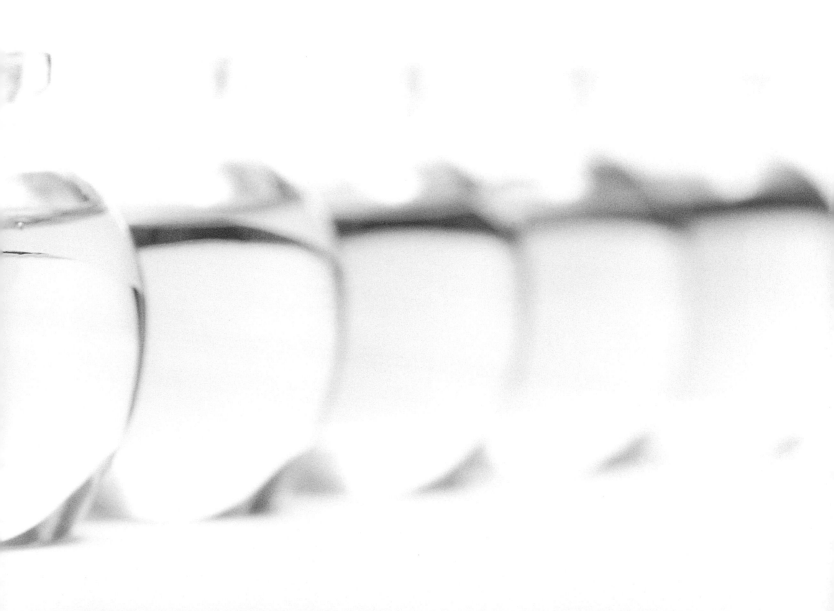

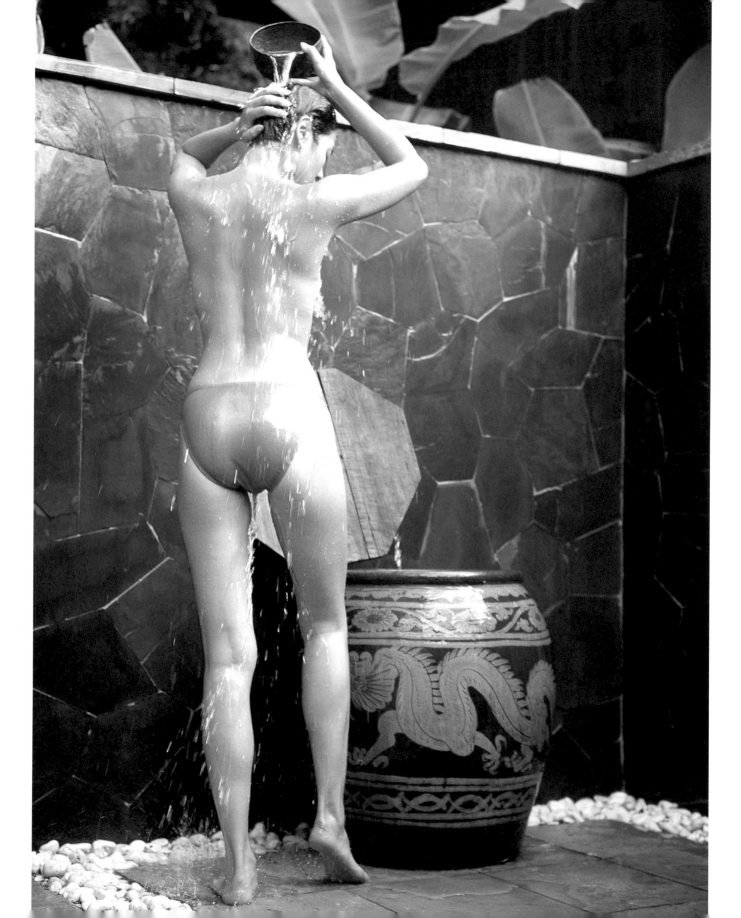

heavenly herbal body treats

Bath and body treatments are some of the therapies that Thai spas excel at. Take the phone off the hook, put on some soothing music and try out some of these popular treatments hot off Thailand's top spa treatment menus; using a variety of traditional ingredients such as medicinal herbs, Thai white mud, essential oils, and native fruits and vegetables, they are guaranteed body bliss-outs.

Baths are an important ritual in Thai life, as Thais bathe frequently to combat the heat of the tropics. Thai settlements were traditionally on the banks of rivers and canals, and houses on stilts faced the waterway, with the entrance marked by a flight of stairs leading up from the water. When bath time came, inhabitants would simply bathe in the river at the bottom of the steps. Little children went naked, while men and women bathed garbed in sarongs, a charming sight along the waterways.

This old-fashioned custom has been adopted by Tamarind Retreat in Koh Samui, where guests are given floral sarongs to wear in the spa. When dipping in the cold-water plunge pool in the rocks, sitting in the natural rock steam room, or having a massage in the open-air pavilion, what could be more comfortable and relaxing than wearing just a cotton sarong between your naked body and the tropical outdoors?

The humid climate, aided by a healthy diet of fresh fruits, herbs and vegetables keeps Thai complexions blissfully moist and wrinkle free. Aside from frequent baths, the sybaritic Thais have devised many ways to keep cool in the heat: *dinsaw* *pong*, or Thai white mud, smeared on the skin and face is a wonderful coolant, and the deodorant stone *saan som* acts as a natural anti-perspirant and deodorant when wetted and rubbed on the skin

Aside from cooling treatments, ancient Thai body treatments included a number of heated healing therapies based on the principles of traditional herbal medicine. Age-old herbal compresses and poultices revive and rejuvenate, and today feature prominently on the Thai spa menu.

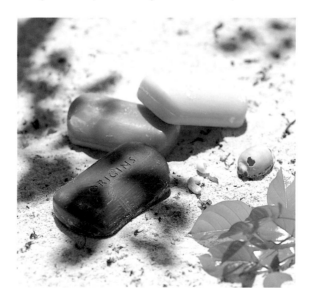

Opposite: In hot weather, there's nothing more refreshing than hefty splashes of cool water — the way Thais used to bathe from rainwater urns in the past.
Left: You don't have to be in Thailand to have a tropical shower. Soaps like these bars from Origins contain essential oils of cloves, menthol, and ylang-ylang. Blended in coconut oil, they smell tropical, but are sold worldwide.

heaven-scented soaks

A soothing, hot bath is a lovely way to comfort tired muscles at the end of a long day. Add some essential oils or a tablespoon of powdered ginger under the tap and let the warm, steamy air work miracles on your body and mind. While you're lying back, close your eyes and put two cooled-in-the-fridge tea bags on them; this will constrict blood vessels and reduce puffiness in the eye area.

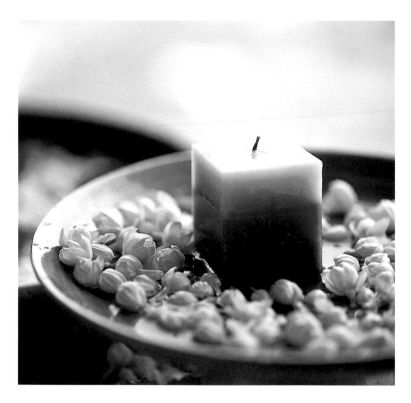

A long soak softens skin and speeds up oil absorption. But if it's a quick pick-me-up you're in need of, take an aromatic shower: Mix some essential oils with a carrier oil, then massage them onto your skin before you get under the shower. Or you can dip a washcloth into the mixture and rub it over your body during the shower. If your shower is in the bathtub, plugging the tub helps the essential oils vaporise in the warm water while you shower.

Try these Thai aromas to wash aches away. Jasmine and tangerine relax and revive after a hard day; ylang-ylang and jasmine are sensuously soothing for a romantic mood; peppermint, lime and basil are a good combo for invigorating a tired body; ginger and eucalyptus ease aches and pains; lime, eucalyptus and tea tree are wonderful for soothing for coughs and colds; tangerine, camphor and ylang-ylang help insomniacs; and a mix of lemongrass, peppermint and lime are reviving hangover cures.

Milk & Honey Purifying Bath

Thais have long believed in the goodness of honey as a medicinal substance that helps cleanse, soothe and moisturise the skin. The Banyan Tree Spa has created a bath of milk and honey to refresh and soften your whole body. Sprinkle some fresh rose petals onto the water just before you step in, and then lie back and enjoy a warm, languorous soak.

3 teaspoons	honey
2 litres	fresh milk
10 drops	your favourite essential oil
1 handful	bath salts
Scattering	red rose petals

Mix the honey, fresh milk and bath salts together and stir well until the honey and bath salts have dissolved. Add the mixture to a tub of warm water. Add the essential oil to the tub, then sprinkle rose petals on the water and luxuriate in a soothing soak.

Five Nectar Bath

For a skin-tingling boost, try the Five Nectar Bath offered by Spa Botanica at the Sukhothai Bangkok. Banana and coconut trees grow all over Thailand, and this nourishing bath uses both. Milk and yoghurt soften the skin, leaving it silky smooth, and honey, used traditionally in Thailand to soften scar tissue on wounds and produced by royal projects under patronage of Her Majesty the Queen, helps to refine pores and slightly lighten the skin.

Pulp	of one banana
2 tablespoons	milk
1 tablespoon	coconut milk
1 tablespoon	yoghurt
1 tablespoon	honey

Mix the ingredients together and massage onto the body. Soak for 10–20 minutes in a warm bath to nourish the skin.

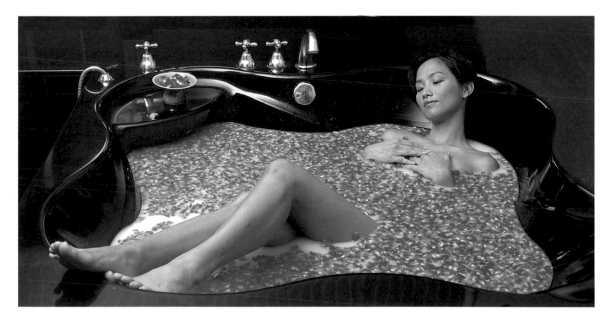

Opposite: Create a romantic mood in your bathroom with an aroma-therapy candle like this one from Angsana Spa. *Left:* Milk baths were luxuries reserved for princesses in the olden days, but now you can make your own. Sprinkle a few rose petals in the bath to give yourself a real royal treat.

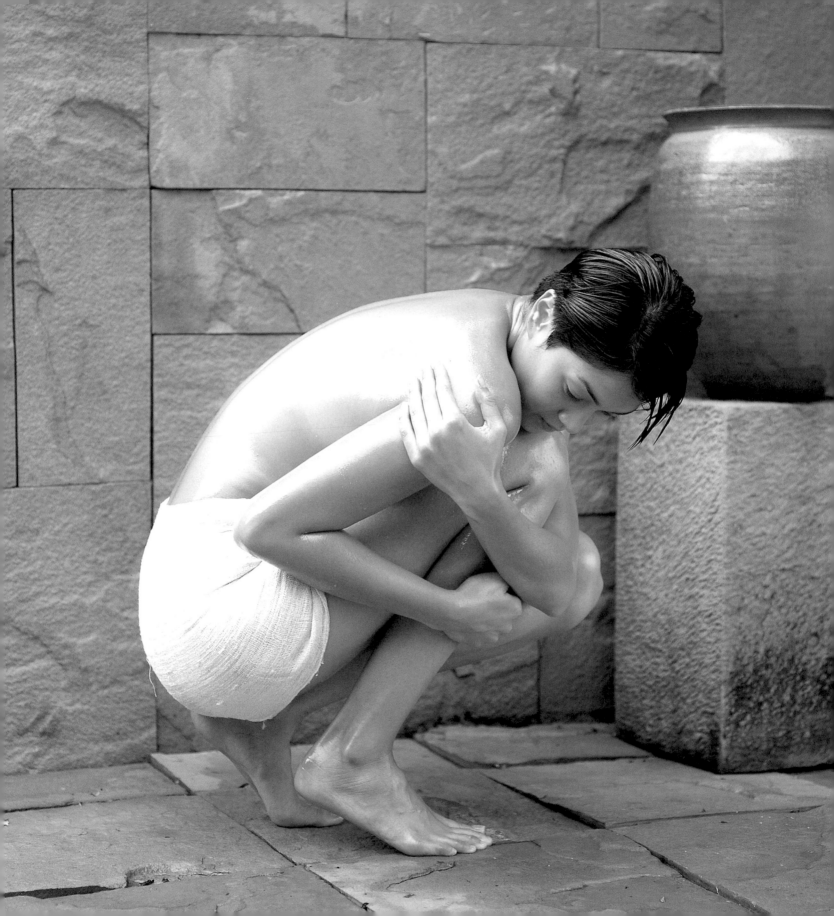

after-bath moisturisers

Since the skin on your arms and legs has few sebaceous glands, your feet, elbows and knees easily become dry and rough without extra moisturising. Moisturising your body is the best and easiest way to pamper your skin. Moisturisers keep skin supple and glowing by sealing the surface of your skin to trap the natural water inside the tissues and stop it from evaporating out into the air.

Essential Oil Moisturiser

An essential oil moisturiser, applied directly after a bath or shower, is one of the most effective do-it-yourself spa treatments. When skin is soft, warm and damp, its rate of absorption is at a premium; it's at this point that oils will most effectively hydrate the skin. Next time you step out of a hot shower or bath, try this seductively simple recipe from The Spa Botanica at the Sukhothai Bangkok, to give you exotically perfumed, sensuously silky skin.

For Mature and Dry Skin

1 tablespoon	almond base oil
2 drops	jasmine essential oil
2 drops	sandalwood essential oil

For All Skin Types

1 tablespoon	almond or jojoba base oil
3 drops	frangipani essential oil

Mix the oils in the palm of your hand and massage all over the body after your shower or bath. Applying the mixture on warm, slightly damp skin helps lock in the moisture.

Egg & Honey Moisturiser

If your skin is dry and dull-looking, you'll want to feed it with egg yolk (high in Vitamin A) and honey — to soothe, cure, soften and enrich the skin. The Banyan Tree Spas in Phuket and Bangkok share their recipe for an at-home body moisturiser that helps to hydrate and improve your skin's texture.

1	egg yolk
1 teaspoon	honey
2 drops	pure olive oil

Mix all the ingredients together and beat well for 2–3 minutes. Spread the mixture all over your body and leave on for 10–15 minutes. Rinse off.

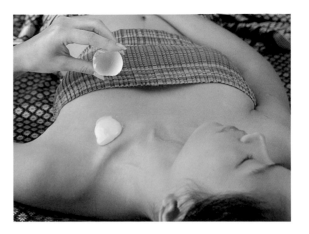

Opposite: The best time to moisturise your body is after a bath, when the warm skin absorbs oils that seal moisture into the damp skin.
Left: Eggs and honey may sound like a dessert recipe, but it's really a nutrient-rich treat for the body, not the tastebuds.

body blasts

Taking their cue from nature, the Thais create a wonderful array of body nourishing recipes for spa and home use. Try any of these body-blasting recipes, for nourishing, revitalizing and protecting the skin.

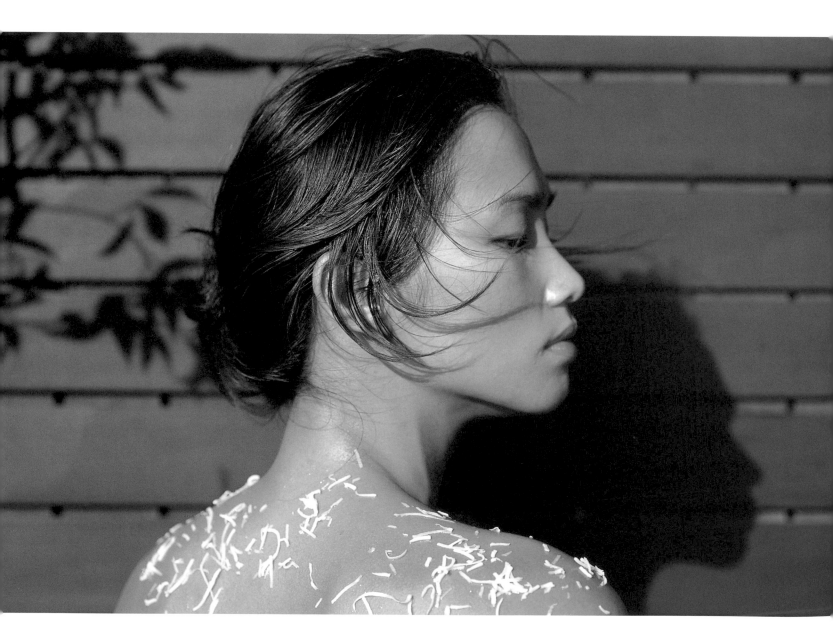

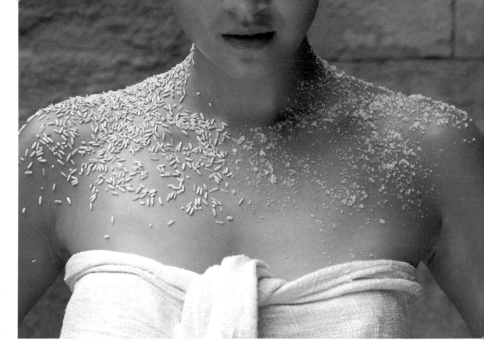

Coconut Pre-Sun Treatment

Coconuts and rice are ubiquitous in Thai landscape and cuisine. Rice is the lifeblood of Thai culture, with important rites and rituals revolving around its cultivation, and the myriad uses of coconut pervade all aspects of Thai life. Taking its cue from the lush growth of coconut trees that dominate the land at Amanpuri Resort, the Aman Spa makes use of the fruit in a luxurious pre-sun body treatment, applied after an aromatherapy massage. Wish you were there? Try recreating the smells and sensations with this simple recipe.

1	coconut
2 tablespoons	ground rice
2 tablespoons	coconut milk

Grate the flesh of the coconut and mix it with the ground rice and coconut milk. Scrub the mixture over your whole body to exfoliate and moisturise the skin, then wrap up in a towel for 10 minutes. Remove the mixture with a warm, damp cloth, then shower off to reveal skin that is soft and smooth to the touch.

Salt Glow Scrub

Though many spas are located on islands or at beach resorts, Le Royal Spa at Le Meridien Phuket Yacht Club offers the rare luxury of outdoor treatment rooms that overlook the sea. You can imagine lying in their sea-view spa when you try their invigorating Salt Glow Scrub.

13 tablespoons	sea salt
300 ml	massage oil of your choice

Mix the ingredients together, then rub the mixture in a circular motion all over the body, starting on legs, then back, arms and stomach. Especially scrub the area around the bikini line and hips, and rough spots on the knees and elbows. Shower off, then apply lotion to moisturise your newly smooth skin.

Opposite: Coconut flesh is rich with oil that gives the skin a silky sheen when rubbed on the body. If you can't find fresh grated coconut, dried coconut soaked in water will do the job as well.
Top: Rice and sea salt have a grainy texture that make them popular ingredients in Thai spa scrubs.

Tamarind Body Scrub

Sun-conscious Thais have used the highly acidic tamarind fruit for centuries as a whitening agent to scrub, exfoliate and polish the skin. Here's a modern day recipe for an age-old beauty treatment, inspired by the tamarind trees that grow in the lush gardens of the Spa Botanica at the Sukhothai Bangkok.

2 tablespoons	tamarind powder
2 tablespoons	rice flour
3–5 drops	neroli essential oil
1 tablespoon	honey

Mix all the ingredients with a little bit of milk until it forms a paste. Massage the paste all over the body, then shower off.

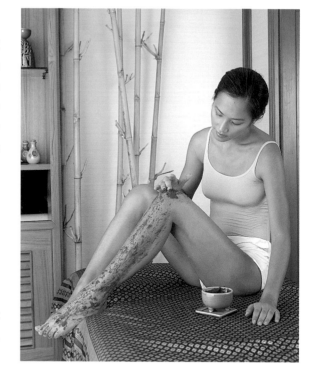

Above: The warming effect of this ginger body scrub is soothing on sore joints and aching muscles — just the right treat for your legs after you've been on your feet all day!
Right: When you can't get to a real spa or make your own scrub, a ready-made mix like this ginger and sea salt scrub from Origins can become part of your bath time routine.
Opposite: This spice mixture may look and smell good enough to eat, but its real benefits are for the skin — massage it on your body and feel how smooth and refreshed it leaves you!

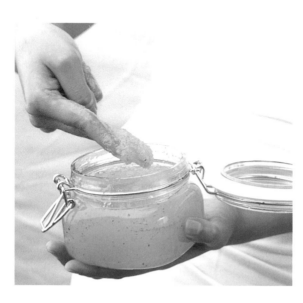

Thai Ginger Body Scrub

The potent ginger rhizome has been widely used by Thais for cooking and healing purposes for centuries. Ginger helps relieve excessive amounts of gas in the stomach and has a warming effect on the body. If your muscles are feeling sore and achy, try rubbing your skin with this home remedy exclusively created by Banyan Tree Spa. The ginger's warmth will penetrate your skin to relieve aching muscles and the rough texture of the rice makes it one of Mother Nature's most effective exfoliants. It is an especially relaxing treat after a strenuous sports activity.

4 tablespoons	ginger powder
4 tablespoons	rice grains
To mix	warm water

Blend the ginger powder and rice grains together, adding a little bit of warm water to dampen the mixture. Apply the mixture in circular, massaging motions all over the body, especially on the joints, muscles or aching areas. Rinse off with warm water in the shower.

Thai Spices Polisher

If you love the spicy aroma of Thai food, you'll enjoy blending this spicy health scrub for your skin. Created by the Angsana Spa Laguna Phuket, this Thai herbal body polisher uses spices that provide antiseptic skin cleansing, soothe the skin, and stimulate blood circulation.

1 teaspoon	Kaffir lime peel powder
1 teaspoon	dry lemongrass, blended
1 teaspoon	cinnamon powder
1 teaspoon	olive oil
2 tablespoons	guava juice

Mix all ingredients together and rub the mixture thoroughly on the whole body in circular, massaging motions, especially working on the rough skin on the elbows and knees. Rinse off with warm water in the shower.

Because the scrub will have sloughed off the dead skin cells on the outer layour of your body, skin tone will be markedly improved. Be sure to moisturise well after.

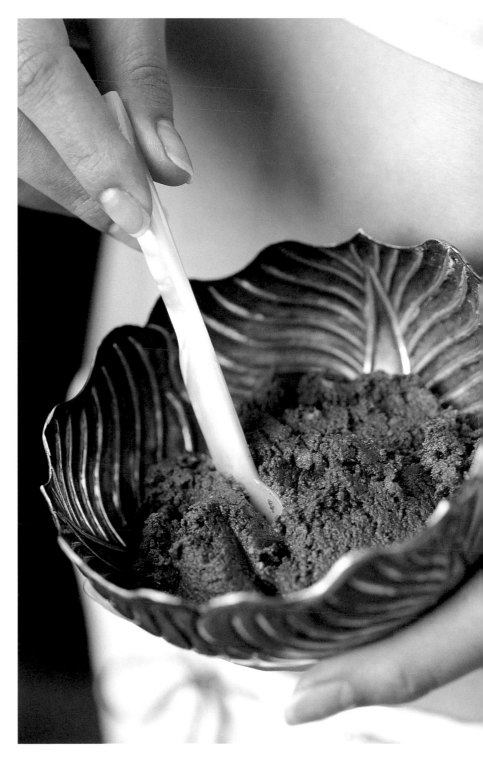

"Modern medical practioners may scoff at the abilities of ancient herbal remedies, but once you experience the healing benefits for yourself, your beliefs change."
— *Khun Komon Chitprasert, traditional therapist and owner, Thai Herbal Spa*

Thai Fruit Body Mask

Thailand's luscious, lovely fruits look good in a basket or on a plate, and if used in the right way, they can make your body look great too! Here, the Regent Chiangmai's Lanna Spa shares an easy recipe for an at-home body treatment to make you feel as fresh and ripe as a Thai fruit salad.

1 cup	plain yoghurt
2 tablespoons	table salt
1 cup	fresh chopped papaya
1 cup	fresh chopped pineapple
1 tablespoon	honey
1 teaspoon	sesame oil
1/2 teaspoon	lemon juice

Right: Body treatment mixtures come in all colours and textures; these skin-savers from the Oriental Spa are (from left to right) Papaya Body Polish, Oriental Herbal Wrap, and Oriental Body Glow. *Opposite:* Fresh papaya is full of vitamins and rich in AHAs. After a papaya body wrap, your skin feels softened and refreshed.

To make the exfoliant, mix the yoghurt and salt in a bowl. For the body mask mixture you need to combine all the remaining ingredients and set aside in a small bowl.

Exfoliate your body by rubbing all over with the yoghurt and salt mixture.

Shower in warm water to rinse off. The salt and yoghurt will open the pores of your skin so the vitamins and nutrients from the mask will be easily absorbed. Apply the body mask mixture over your entire body and leave on for 20 minutes. Rinse off in a warm shower, and apply body lotion. The skin will be soft, silky and have a natural glow.

Papaya Body Polish

The deep, rich orange colour of Thai papayas gives you a mere visual hint of the fruit's succulent sweet flesh that is bursting with vitamins C and A. Not just a treat for the tastebuds and the eyes, papaya is known to be rich in AHAs, the Alpha Hydroxy Acids naturally occurring in fruits that help exfoliate the skin. This fruit is a popular and effective ingredient in body wrap treatments to polish and smoothen the complexion.

Simply mash the flesh of a ripe papaya to a pulp. Massage the mixture all over the body, and wrap in a plastic sheet for 15 minutes. Rinse off to reveal soft, moistened skin.

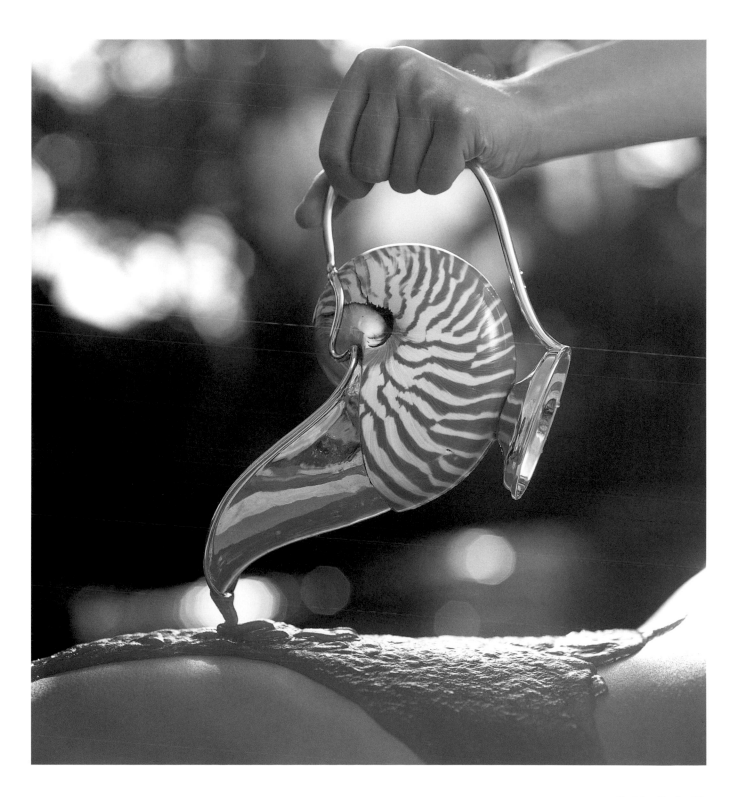

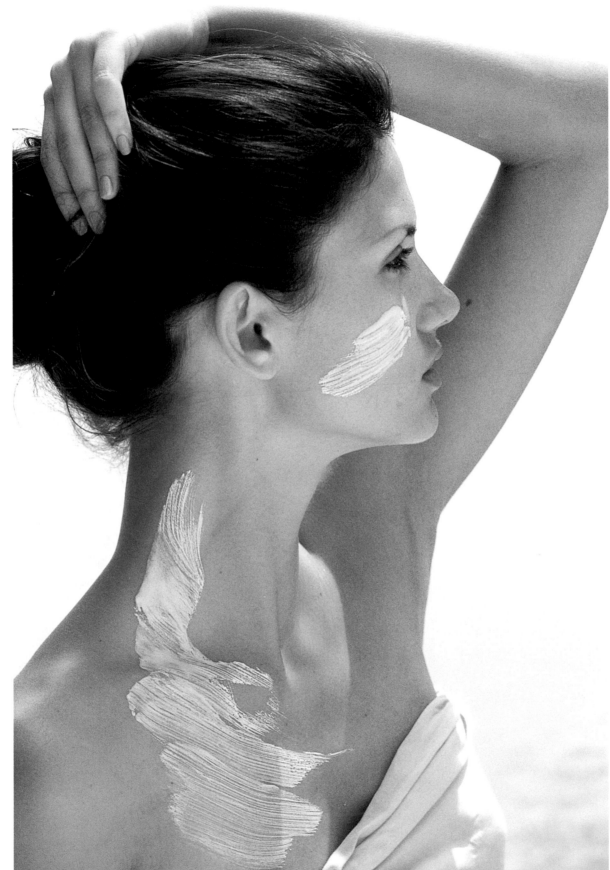

Opposite and right: Thai white mud is nature's sunblock. Simply mix it with water to form a thick paste that gives instant relief and protection from the sun's burning effects. In modern day Thai spa treatments, *dinsaw pong* is used as an ingredient in face masks and body wraps for its cooling and healing properties, as well as to soften skin.

beat the heat

Rich, smooth, earthy, and sensuous, mud has served as nature's sunblock in hot, humid climates for generations. A coat of cool, wet mud provides welcome relief from the relentless heat of the tropics, and with the right kind of mud, a mineral-rich mud body mask can draw out impurities and act as a natural healing remedy for rashes and irritated skin. Sun-seekers should check these recipes out.

Jungle Rain Body Mask

The torrential downpours of the Asian monsoon are another of nature's body-coolers, but monsoon lasts only part of the year. So if you're stuck in a heat wave, you can enjoy this luxurious body treatment. The Spa Botanica's Jungle Rain Mask body treatment uses cooling green clay to help absorb impurities, cleanse the pores and exfoliate the skin, while a combination of the essential oils of *prai*, cedarwood and mandarin create an uplifting and positive mood for mind and spirit.

3 tablespoons	green mud powder
2 tablespoons	avocado oil
3 tablespoons	aloe vera
2 drops each	essential oil of *prai*, cedarwood and mandarin

You will need two dishes, a small one for the oil and a bigger one for the green mud powder. Mix the essential oils into the avocado oil first, then mix this into the green mud powder and add the aloe vera. Stir till it becomes an even paste, diluting with water until it is the consistency of cake mix. Apply on the body, leave on for 20 minutes, then rinse off.

Thai White Mud

The Thais have their own indigenous version, a native clay known as Thai white mud, or *dinsaw pong*, that has been used as a cooling and healing natural body treatment for centuries. Not really a mud, but more like a thick white chalk, it effervesces in water. It has a pleasant smell and in olden times the loose clay was used in the same manner as talc after a shower, to help cool the body.

Dinsaw pong is readily available in the form of white triangular pellets in Thailand. To use it in the Thai traditional manner, simply dissolve the pellets in water, and smear the paste on the face and body as a natural skin cooler and protector.

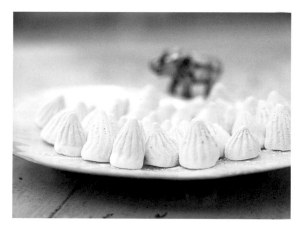

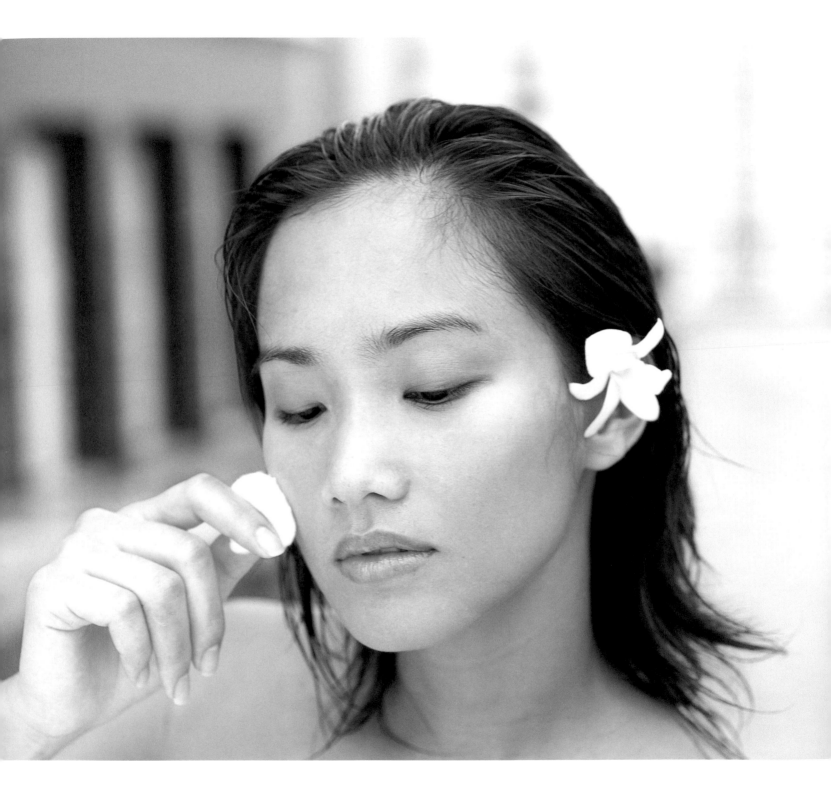

saving face

Thais are easy-going by nature and smile for any reason or no apparent reason at all. They seem to look years younger than their actual age and don't have many wrinkles, perhaps because they enjoy life with happy-go-lucky abandon. This attitude is aptly expressed in the oft-used phrases *'mai pen wrai'* ('never mind'), *'sabai, sabai'* ('relax, relax'), and *'jai yen, yen'* ('keep a cool heart') — positive internal attitudes that manifest themselves on their cheerful faces. Similarly, Thai people have an inherent sense of *sanook* or fun, radiating inner good feelings in the form of serene, smiling faces.

The idea of *sabai, sabai* is inherent in the Thai spa: exotic scents, gentle sounds and welcoming smiles immediately put one at ease — and frown lines, tension and anxiety that unconsciously show on the face start to disappear. And of course, after a stress-busting, pampering spa treatment, you'll feel like smiling both inside and out.

As in most Asian cultures, fair skin is prized among Thais and the key concern of Thai women is to avoid the damaging, darkening effects of the sun. Face-saving, traditional beauty treatments were aimed at whitening the complexion and protecting it from tanning and sunburn. Since the humid tropical climate tended to keep the skin moist most of the time, creams to prevent wrinkles were not prevalent. Try some of the following Thai-and-tested treatments to relax, rejuvenate and promote a fair complexion.

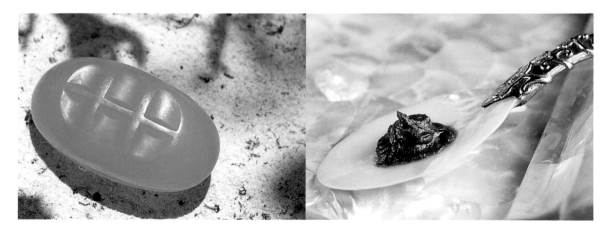

Far left: Gylcerine soaps are pure and gentle on sensitive complexions. This tangerine-scented bar from Origins can be uplifting as well as cleansing!
Left: The highly acidic tamarind fruit has been used as a skin brightening cosmetic by centuries of Thai women. Traditional herbal preparations like this one can be bought over the counter in Thai herbal shops.

immaculate complexions

For centuries Thais have looked to nature for healing and nourishing therapies. On many Thai spa menus today, you'll find treatments that use traditional complexion-enhancing ingredients, even if they are no longer found in modern-day cosmetics.

Certain native fruits like tamarind and lime were used as whitening agents because their high acidity made them effective exfoliants, ridding the complexion of dead surface cells and revealing the fresh new skin beneath. Watermelon and papaya are good exfoliators too. Also, certain plants were known for their ability to beautify and nourish the skin: *prai* has been used by Thais for centuries as a skin softener, while healing turmeric clears the skin and the ivy gourd leaf (*tumleung*) moisturises and nourishes. For sunburn, try aloe vera, cucumber and Thai white mud (*dinsaw pong*). Alternatively try some of these simple recipes courtesy of the Mandara Spa.

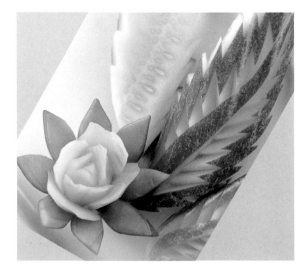

Right: With its high water content, raw chilled cucumber can provide moisturising relief for your face on a hot day. *Opposite:* Called the 'crocodile tail plant' in Thai, aloe vera flesh is a refreshing natural gel that is one of nature's best beauty ingredients to cool sunburn and moisturise skin.

Fruity and Floral Face Toners

Fruits and vegetables are not only good to eat, but they also contain vitamins and enzymes that have the ability to soothe, tone and exfoliate the skin. These facial toners are all natural and very refreshing. Take your pick of any of the following ingredients; one ingredient makes one toner.

Aloe Vera — nourishing, for all skin types
Cucumber — toning, for oily skin
Guava — exfoliating, with natural AHA
Lemongrass — cleansing, for all skin types
Pineapple — exfoliating, with natural AHA
Tamarind — exfoliating and whitening, for oily skin
Tomato — moisturising, for all skin types

Use 50 grams per ingredient. Wash, dry, peel and blend the ingredients in a food processor. Mix with 25 ml (¼ cup) distilled water and allow the solution to settle. Strain and discard the solid particles.

The remaining solution can be used as a fresh toner. Apply some of the liquid to a cotton wool pad and rub gently all over the face after cleansing. Depending on which solution you have chosen, your complexion will either be cleansed, toned, nourished or all three.

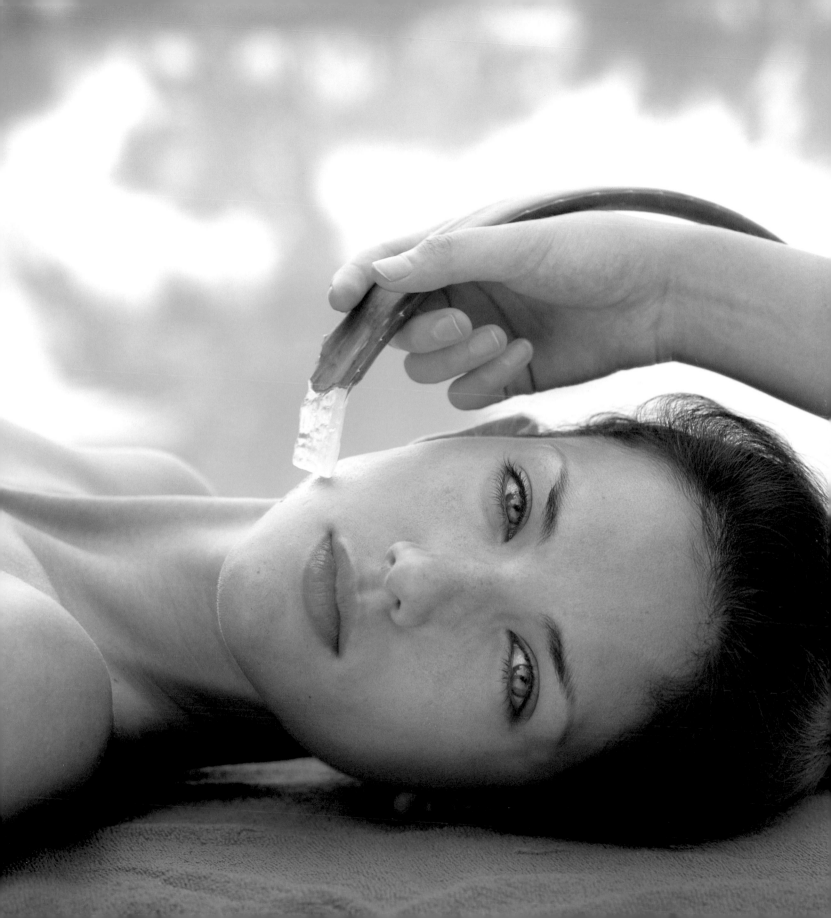

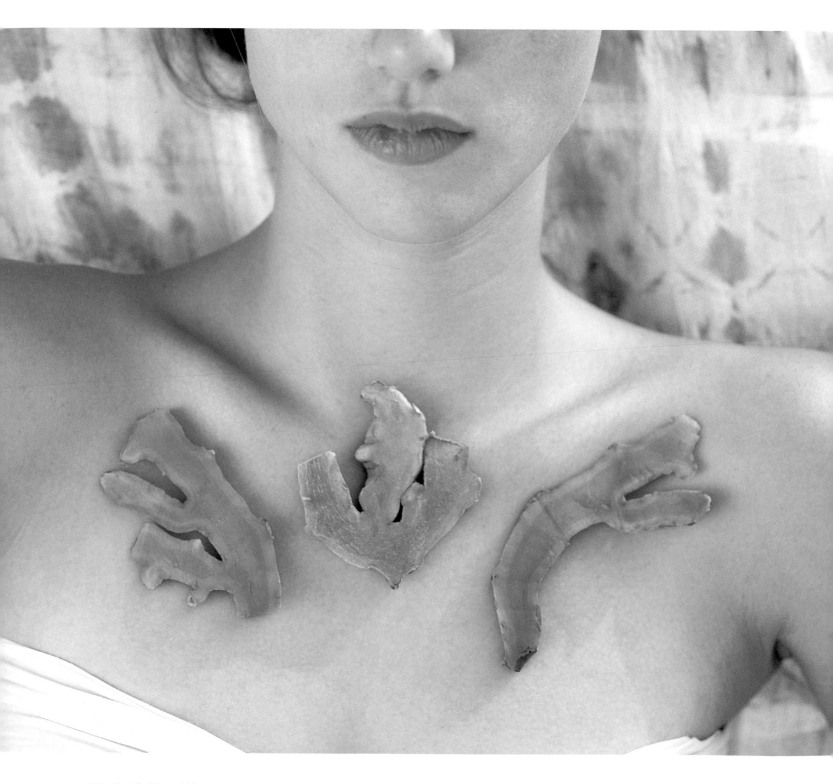

Turmeric Face Mask

Turmeric has long been used by Thais for its anti-inflammatory and healing properties to help cleanse and clear up the complexion. Soybean contains estrogen, progesterone and phyto estrogen, and is used as a skin whitener and softener. In the olden times this recipe would have been made using an old-fashioned mortar and pestle, but with a kitchen blender, it's a no-nonsense beauty treatment that can be made in next to no time at all.

10 g	fresh turmeric
15 g	soybeans

Wash, peel, and blend the turmeric in a good food processor. Set the pulp aside. Soak the soybeans for 20 minutes, then blend them and mix in with the turmeric to make a paste. Spread the mixture evenly on the face, leave it for 10 minutes, then wash off with warm water.

Banana and Jasmine Face Reviver Mask

This mineral-rich face mask from the Regent Chiangmai's Lanna Spa uses Thailand's ever abundant bananas and sweet smelling jasmine flowers to revive and refresh your face after a long and tiring day. Bananas are rich in vitamin A and potassium and the jasmine essential oil enhances skin toning and helps to prevent scarring. Wheat germ oil and honey are hydrating and nourishing.

2	ripe bananas, medium size
½ teaspoon	wheat germ oil
2 teaspoons	honey
2 drops	jasmine oil

Mash the bananas and combine with the remaining ingredients in a bowl, mixing well with a spatula. Cleanse and tone your face, then apply the mixture in circular motions. Leave the mixture on the face for 20 minutes, then rinse off with warm water and tone again to remove any residue.

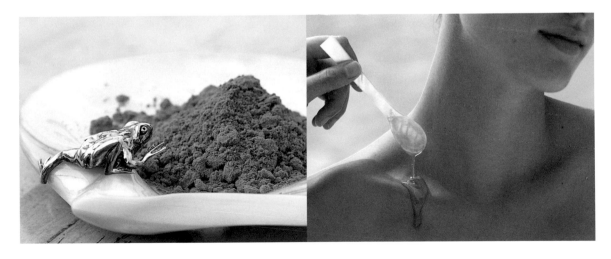

Opposite and far left: Raw turmeric resembles its cousin, ginger on the outside, but when sliced reveals a bright orange flesh with a sharp, earthy smell. Dried, powdered turmeric is used in herbal pastes for the face and body.
Left: Honey is humectant and leaves skin feeling nourished and soft.

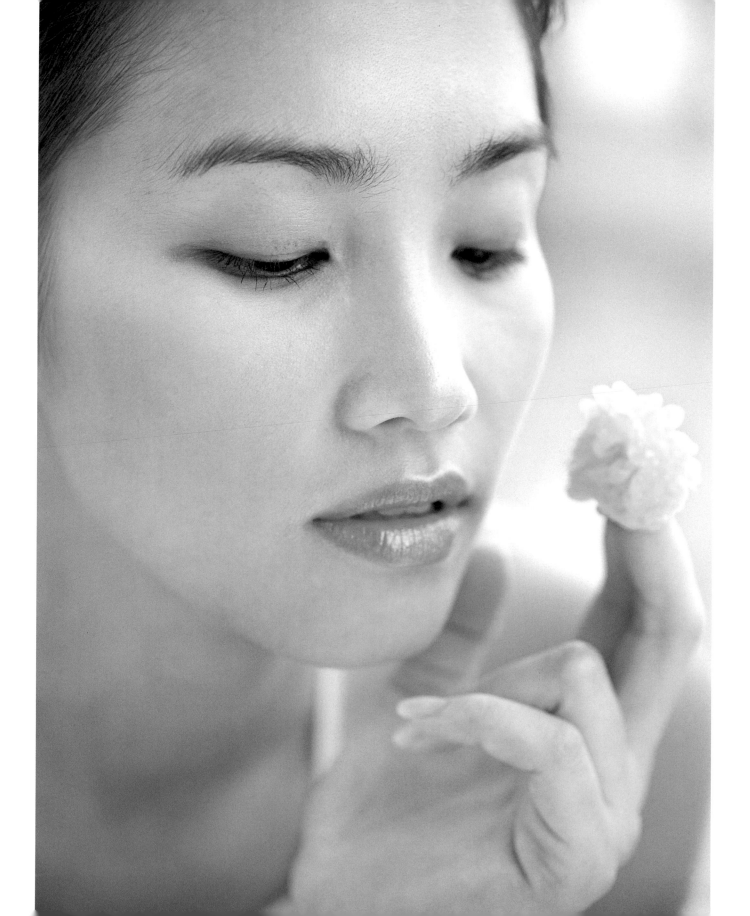

Honey & Tangerine Facelift

Known for its healing and anti-bacterial properties, honey has been used by many cultures, including Thailand, in herbal remedies for centuries. The Banyan Tree Spa uses honey with oranges and lavender essential oil in a quick-fix mask that leaves the face soft and glowing. This is a mild treatment that can be done regularly to improve the texture of the skin and lighten blemishes.

1 piece	orange or tangerine
1 teaspoon	honey
1 drop	lavender essential oil

Rub the piece of orange all over the face. The fruit acid helps to cleanse while providing moisture to plump up fine lines. Gently wipe off the face with a natural sponge or muslin cloth dipped in warm water. Mix the honey with lavender essential oil and apply the mixture to the face by massaging lightly. Leave the mixture on for 5–10 minutes, then rinse off with warm water.

Facial Scrub

You'll be surprised by how many of the ingredients of your fridge or store cupboard can double up as a kitchen cosmetic. And it's a fun way to spend the afternoon, concocting different pastes and solutions for an at-home facial. A root of the ginger family, *prai* has a distinctive aroma and is cherished by Thais as a panacea for the skin. It is a popular ingredient in moisturising and nourishing skin treatments and is often found in massage oils. This simple face scrub is suitable for all skin types, and smells exotically spicy too.

I tablespoon	fresh *prai*
I teaspoon	nutmeg powder

Wash, dry, peel, then pulp the turmeric in a blender. Squeeze out the liquid and set aside the pulp. Mix the fresh turmeric pulp with nutmeg powder until you get a paste. Gently scrub the mixture all over your face, then rinse off.

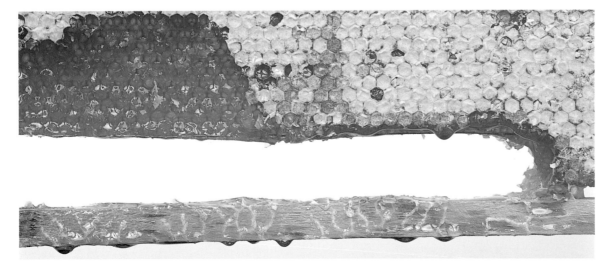

Left: Honey has long been famed for its anti-bacterial properties that improve the skin's texture, but the secret is to use pure, fresh honey for maximum effectiveness.

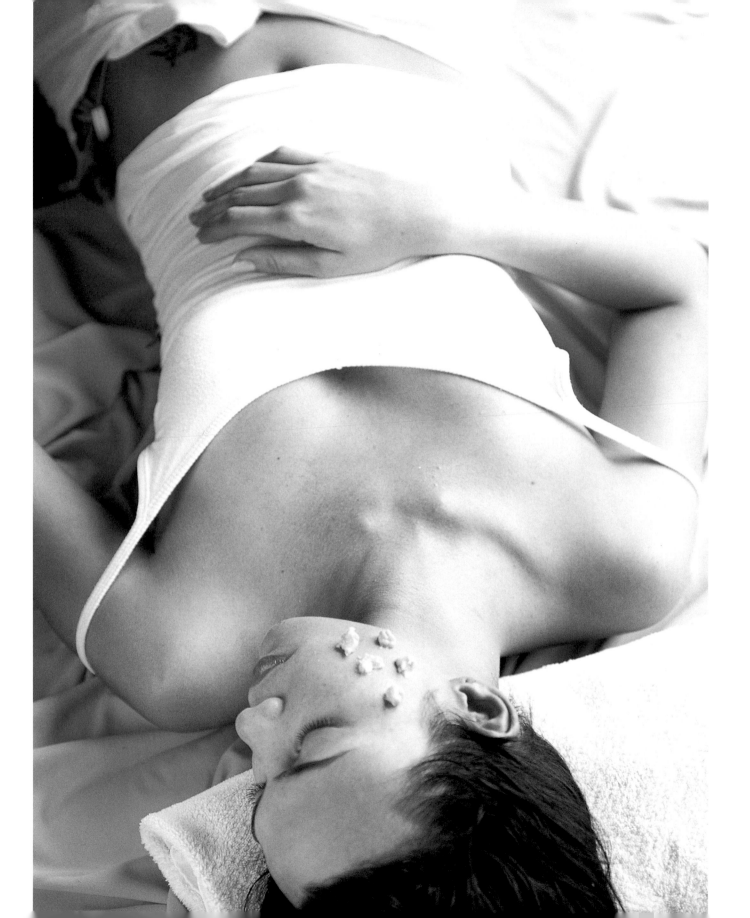

"Always remember to smile to yourself. Smiling beautifies your face, but when you bring the smile inside your heart and mind, you beautify your whole being."
— *Mae-Chee Sansanee, founder of Santhira-Dhammasthan Ashram, Bangkok*

Banana & Avocado Face Mask for Dry Skin

Thailand's great variety of sweet bananas find their way into most Thai desserts, but few people are aware that these abundantly common fruits also make effective moisturisers for the face. Bananas are full of potassium and contain rich natural oils along with Vitamins A, B, C and E, that give elasticity to the skin. Combined with the vitamin and mineral-rich, moisturising properties of avocado, the result is a creamy, smooth and deliciously scented mask to add suppleness to your complexion.

1	small ripe banana
1	small ripe avocado
2 tablespoons	plain natural yoghurt
2 drops	Vitamin E Oil

Mash the banana and avocado together to form a thick, lime-green coloured paste. Add the yoghurt and Vitamin E oil and mix well.

Clean and gently steam your face under a towel and over a bowl of boiling water. Then massage the mixture on your face and leave it on for 15 minutes. This mask can be left on for up to 25 minutes though for very sensitive skin, 10 minutes is enough. Rinse off to reveal a refreshed and moisturised face.

Fragrant Face Tonics

Thai flowers are known for their sensuous aromas, but what is less known is that many also have medicinal properties. These flowers are not only fragrant, but make delightful toners suitable for all skin types. One ingredient makes one toner.

Petals of Jasmine, White Orchid, Rose or Champak

Use 50 grams per ingredient. Wash, dry, peel and blend the ingredients in a food processor. Mix with 50 ml (½ cup) distilled water and let the solution settle. Strain and discard the solid particles. Use the remaining solution as a refreshing toner to make you smell and look beautiful.

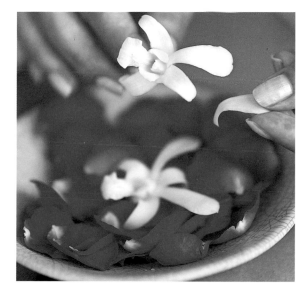

Left: Thai white orchids are not only decorative — they have medicinal properties that can enhance your complexion as well.

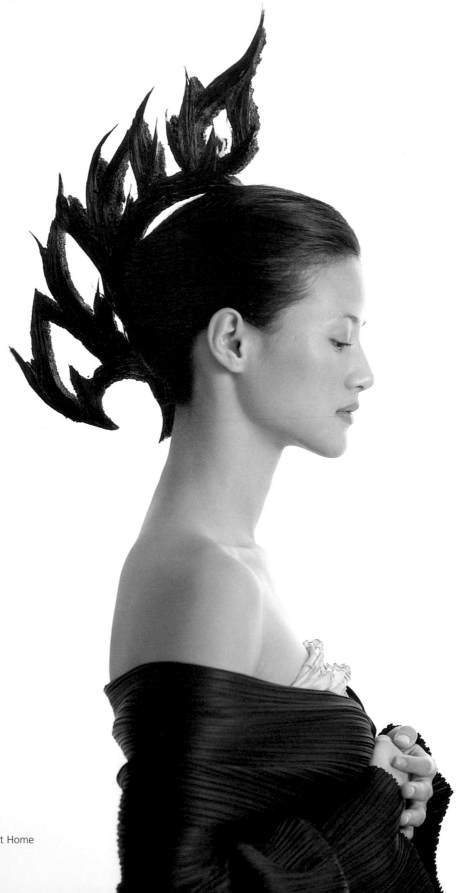

This elaborate hairpiece is a high-fashion fantasy crafted from real hair. The flame-shaped design reproduces the classic Thai pattern found on paintings and temple carvings — a distinctly Thai design motif that makes a fabulous modern hairstyle as well!

healthy hair

Traditionally in Thailand, the darker and shinier the hair, the more prized it was for its beauty. To this end, the Thais have harvested flowers, herbs, seeds and roots — and concocted a plethora of beauty-enhancing hair treatments. In fact, it is precisely because Thai women have relied on nature's yield that their hair looks so sleek and shiny.

Hair is weighted with symbolism in Thai culture. It played an important role in life's rites and rituals, as well as in the country's history. Prior to the 18th century both Thai men and women kept their hair long and lush, usually worn in a topknot on top of the head. However, for special occasions, a number of highly elaborate, sculptural styles were conceived, but these are rarely seen today (see left). Towards the end of the magnificent Ayutthya period, around the 18th century, Thai people began to keep their hair crew-cut short, a style that sprang from the warring incursions from neighbouring Burma. The idea was that a population with hair short, and thus maintenance-free, would be ready to take up arms and defend their country from invaders at any moment.

Though hardly flattering, this short crop remained the national hairstyle until the 20th century, when western fashions were introduced by King Chulalongkorn, who learned from his travels in Europe that short hair on women was deemed unattractive in the west. His queens were the first to start growing their hair long again, thus setting the trend for fashionable society.

This opened the door again for the resurrection of a variety of herbal treatments that had been used by Thai women to keep their tresses glossy and lustrous. A favourite was the dark purple butterfly pea flower (see page 16 and 115), which, when soaked in water, produces a gorgeous, deep blue coloured rinse. It kept hair dark and healthy, and was used to keep gray hair at bay.

The delightfully fragrant soap nut is another ancient Thai ingredient used for nourishing the hair. When crushed and mixed in water, this nut produces a foam that was used for washing the hair and face, and is known to cure dandruff and give the hair a silky sheen, not to mention enhance the tresses with its rich, woodsy-spicy smell. Kaffir lime is another age-old ingredient in traditional hair treatments, esteemed by Thais for its ability to remove dandruff, cleanse the scalp and leave hair shiny and soft.

Some spas in Thailand have taken creative new approaches to beautiful hair, using both age-old remedies as well as their own combinations of new ingredients. Read on for a few of their easy-to-try hair treatments for a healthy, herbal head.

in tip-top condition

Think of conditioning as the final yet essential step in proper haircare. What could be gentler and more nourishing than nature's rich ingredients to add life to your locks? Try these all-natural treatments for shine and bounce — the two signals of healthy, sleek hair.

Sensual Scented Conditioner

You'll find the air perfumed with the luxurious scents of Thai flowers when strolling through the gardens of the Spa Botanica, Thailand's only spa based around a garden concept. Among the flowers in the spa garden, two have been used in their recipe for an oil hair conditioner that soothes the scalp. Ylang-ylang has an intense aroma and because it is night-scented, can only be picked in the early hours; and jasmine is very often seen braided in Asian tresses because of its sweet smell. Try this recipe — your hair will smell like a tropical garden afterwards!

5–10 tbsp	coconut oil (depending on hair length)
8 drops	ylang-ylang essential oil (for oily scalp and hair) or
6 drops	jasmine essential oil (for dry scalp and hair)

Mix the ingredients together. Shampoo and towel dry hair, then apply the mixture, massaging into the scalp and hair. For additional absorption wrap a hot towel around the head. Leave the mixture on for at least 20 minutes, then rinse and shampoo out.

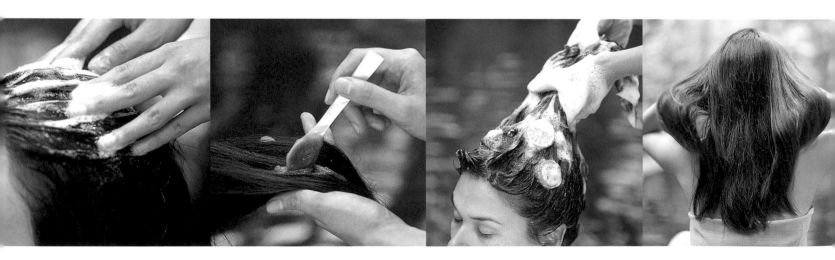

"Thais have always believed in the power of fresh Kaffir lime as a natural beauty ingredient to make hair shine and cure dandruff — it is fairly simple to apply and smells so refreshing too."
— *Shelley Poplak, director, Tamirind Retreat*

Kaffir Lime Hair Conditioner

Kaffir lime has long been cherished as nature's remedy for beautiful, healthy hair. Traditionally, the Thais cut the fruit in half and rubbed it directly onto the hair. The refreshing juice and oil from the fruit's warty skin helped to prevent against dandruff and hair loss, and the tresses were left silky soft.

This recipe comes from the Banyan Tree Spa in Phuket and Bangkok as an easy home remedy to give you citrus-fresh hair. Banyan Tree try to use as many natural ingredients as possible in their treatments, believing that nature is often — if not always — best.

1	Kaffir lime
2 tablespoons	fresh aloe vera

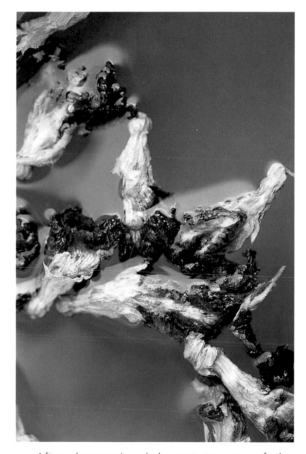

Break off the tail end of the aloe vera leaf and wash this piece thoroughly. Then peel off the skin and mix the aloe vera in a blender. Set aside 2 tablespoons of the blended aloe vera for further mixing. Cut the Kaffir lime into quarters. Blend the pieces with a little bit of water and strain the mixture. Mix the Kaffir lime juice with the freshly prepared aloe vera, stirring until a fairly thick paste has been achieved.

After shampooing (why not try one of the herbal Butterfly Pea flower shampoos readily available in Bangkok stores?) apply the mixture on the hair. Leave it on for 10–15 minutes, then rinse off with cold water.

hair treats

A shampoo's job is to clean your hair and scalp, and a conditioner's job is to moisturise and nourish. Dull, dry hair may be a sign of poor diet or weak health, but even healthy hair can become stripped of its natural moisture by harsh ingredients in chemical-laden hair products or from processing. Try some of these all-herbal hair treats for stunning results.

Egg and Olive Hair Mask

Thai girls have long been advised to treat dry and unhealthy hair with raw egg yolk. This treatment from the Angsana Spa Laguna Phuket incorporates the nutritious egg yolk with olive oil and honey to give you an excellent remedy for dry and dull hair. It leaves hair soft, with a healthy shine.

2	raw egg yolks (more for longer hair)
3 teaspoons	warm olive oil
3 teaspoons	honey

Mix all the ingredients together and massage the mixture well into the hair and scalp. Wrap hair with a towel and leave the mask on for 15–20 minutes. Rinse off with warm water.

Exotic Hair Thickening Rinse

This aromatic rinse from the Spa Botanica can be used to treat either oily or normal hair. Ylang-ylang is said to help increase hair growth and is soothing for irritated and oily skin. If you have an oily scalp, use this hair rinse every second day. Not only is mint antiseptic and gives a cooling effect to the scalp, it combats dandruff and stimulates hair growth as well.

1 cup	warm water
6 drops	ylang-ylang essential oil (for oily scalp and hair)
	or
6 drops	mint essential oil (for normal scalp and hair)

Just before you step in the shower, add the ylang-ylang or mint essential oil to the warm water. Shampoo and condition your hair, then apply the hair rinse.

Opposite: The basic bun was the classic hairstyle for both Thai men and women in the olden days. These days it's an elegant solution for unwashed hair. Here, the bun imitates art, echoing this painting by Thai artist Natee Utarit entitled 'Karanee' in which the artist explores the relationship between the abstract and the realistic.

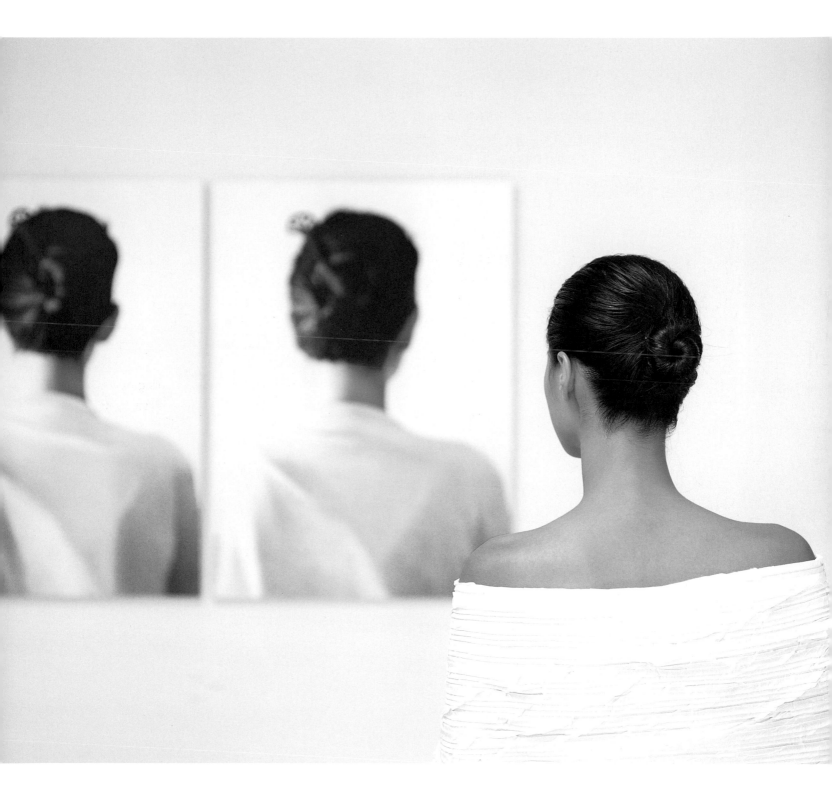

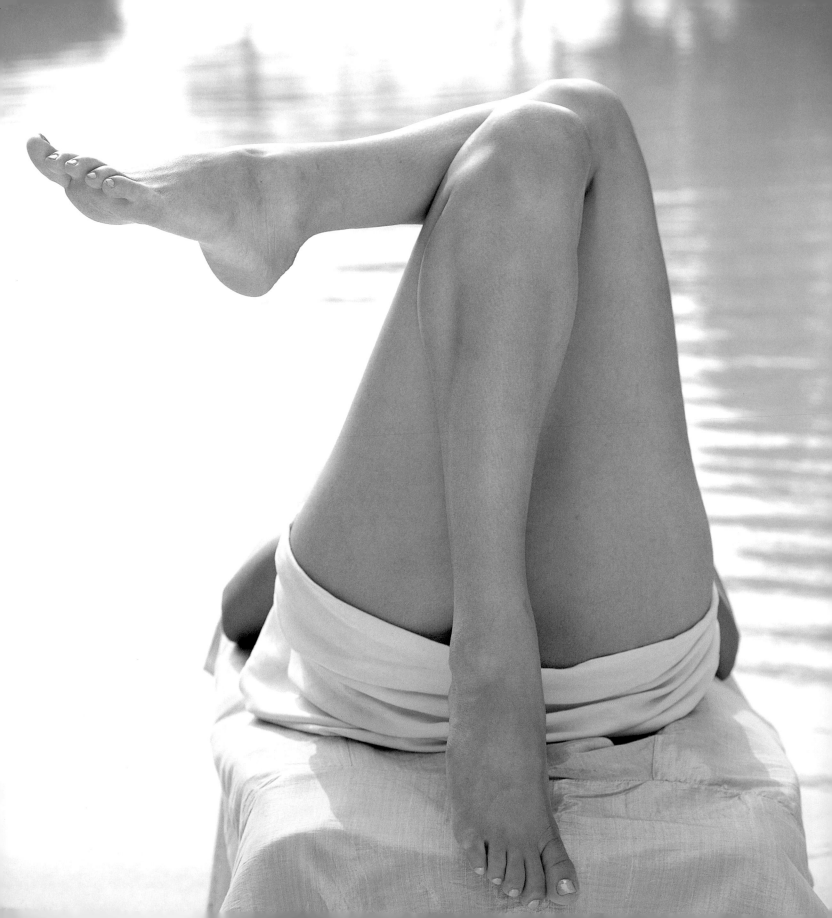

barefoot bliss

Going barefoot is second nature to Thais. Historically, Thai people never wore shoes until the 20th century, when modernising influences brought western fashions and customs to the country. Up until then, the majority of the population padded around on the soft earth, unshod in tropical bliss.

Thai houses were (and often still are) raised on stilts, and every house had an urn of water with a ladle at the foot of the entrance stairs, for cleaning the feet before entering the home. Traditionally, all domestic activities such as sitting, eating, and sleeping took place on the smooth wooden floor, which was kept meticulously clean. These days, modern western furniture replaces the soft reed mats that used to keep people cool and comfortable on the floor, but the custom of honouring the sanctity of the home by leaving shoes at the door remains one of the most important aspects of Thai etiquette.

Some Thai spas have adopted this custom as well. At the Oriental Spa in Bangkok, where the spa interior is meant to convey the sense of a teak panelled, traditional Thai house, guests are asked to remove their shoes at the entrance, as if they are entering a Thai home. The Regent Chiangmai Resort's Lanna Spa is inspired by the concept of a Thai temple, and when guests enter the ante-chamber leading to the spa entrance, shoes come off as they would upon entering a sacred place.

Thais are most comfortable in their bare feet, but would shudder at the thought of kicking back and putting their feet up, in the western sense.

Using one's foot to point, especially at another person, is considered the height of rudeness in Thailand, because the feet are the lowest and most offensive part of the body, and the head the highest and most sacred. Thus, the traditional sitting posture for Thai women is on the floor, leaning on one hip with both legs tucked demurely under one side of the body, pointing away from the person they are facing. The result is a sinuously sexy silhouette.

People who live in the tropics generally enjoy the luxury of healthy feet from walking barefoot on wooden floors, fresh grass or beach sand. Going barefoot means the feet don't suffer the indignity of corns and bunions from being trapped in shoes all the time. But Thais still understand the need to pamper the feet because, with their roots as an agricultural society, who would better know the joy of a relaxing foot massage after a long day of toiling in the fields? That's why Thai massage always starts with the feet: they bear the body's weight and it's where the body's aches and pains accumulate.

These days Thai spas take foot pampering to another level, with a variety of treatments to refresh, revive, and invigorate sore and tired feet. Inspired by traditional ingredients and therapies, they share some of their latest foot treatments.

Opposite: You'll be eager to put your best foot forward when your legs look this fabulous! The skin on your legs and feet are prone to dryness, so keep them moisturised with vegetable oil-based moisturisers that are more easily absorbed into the skin than mineral oils.

feet first

Most of us don't give much thought to our feet unless we're buying shoes — or they're giving us problems! You may not realise it, but your feet are subject to all manner of stresses during the course of the day, from supporting your body, to being confined in tight shoes or twisted in high heeled pumps — which is why at the end of the day you may suffer from sore, aching feet. Your feet can benefit from pampering as much as the rest of your body, and the best way to start is by keeping them moisturised to look and feel their lovely best. Here we give you a few remedies to revive and rejuvenate tired toes.

Banana & Honey Night Cream

Healthy feet are strong and flexible, with natural shock absorbers built into the ball of the foot and the heel, and toes that provide balance for the whole body. However, they need to be treated with respect with regular pedicures, well-fitting shoes, and plenty of little treats. If they're tired, try this natural home remedy created by the Banyan Tree Spa, Phuket. All you need are the contents of your fridge! Honey's humectant properties nourish and moisturise, the banana is soft and soothing, and the lime is an antiseptic.

half	ripe banana
one teaspoon	honey
half teaspoon	lime juice

Mash the banana and mix all the ingredients well, then apply the mixture all over your feet before going to bed. Put on a pair of cotton socks and leave on overnight. You'll wake up to find smoother and softer feet.

Lime Foot Freshener

Lime is an essential ingredient in every Thai kitchen, and this citrus quick fix washes the dull skin off your feet while giving them a fragrant pick-me-up too. The Angsana Spa Laguna Phuket offers a comprehensive, 90-minute foot treatment of foot cleansing and wrapping in their outdoor pavilions, but here they share a quick and easy treatment to re-create the Thai spa experience at home.

4 slices	lime
1 teaspoon	lime juice
1 teaspoon	brown sugar

Thoroughly mix the lime juice and brown sugar and set aside. Put the lime slices in a large basin filled with warm water. Soak your feet in the water for about 10–15 minutes. Rinse off with warm water and dry with a clean towel. Gently scrub the lime juice and brown sugar mixture on the feet in circular motions, particularly on the hardened skin areas around the heels. Rinse off with warm water.

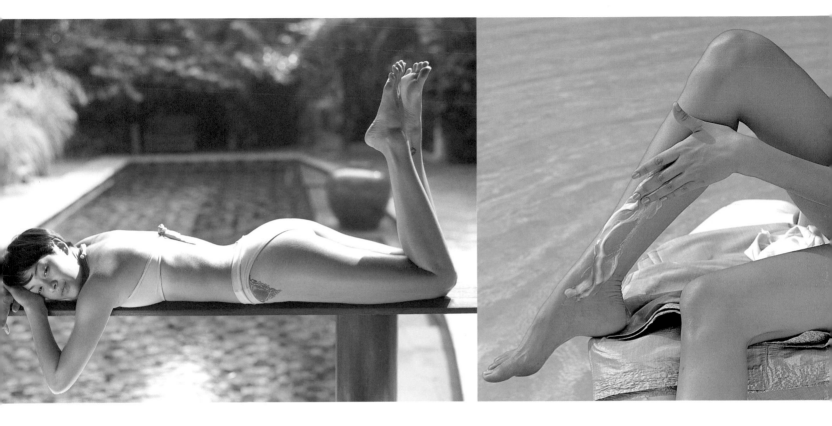

Hydrating Extremity Ritual

The rhizome *prai* has long been used by Thais as a natural moisturiser that helps to nourish and soften the skin. Here, *prai* and coconut feature in the Regent Chiangmai's Lanna Spa deep-moisturising recipe to remedy dry feet

1 tablespoon	*prai* oil
1 tablespoon	coconut oil
1 tablespoon	sesame oil
1 teaspoon	vitamin E oil
1 teaspoon	honey
½ tablespoon	glycerin preparation

Put the honey into a saucepan and bring to a simmer until it becomes runny. Stir constantly and watch that it does not burn, then turn the ring down to low. Add the oil, Vitamin E and glycerin, stir until thoroughly mixed, then let the mixture cool to room temperature.

Before going to bed, apply the rich, hydrating and nourishing oil onto your feet and toenails, massaging the mixture in for several minutes. Put on a pair of cotton socks and leave on overnight. There should be some leftover mixture that you can put in a jar and use the following day. You'll awaken with smooth, firm and toned looking feet!

essentially delightful dips

If you've been on your feet all day and feel completely beat, a soothing foot soak is the best reward for worn out feet. It warms and relaxes all the tiny support muscles in your feet, releases trapped nerves, improves the blood circulation and soothes aches and pains.

Sole-soothing Scents

Adding the right essential oil makes a foot bath a completely pampering experience. It's the healing properties of the essential oils that effect the improvements in the way you feel. All you need is a large basin, hot water, a towel, a comfortable seat, and the essential oils. Add the oils drop by drop as you slide your feet in the water, about one drop to one litre (2.2 pints) of water.

To make the whole experience more seductive, throw in some flower petals as well. Just the sight of some frangipani blooms or rose petals tingling the tips of your toes will help you put your best foot forward afterwards.

Try any of these oils for instant relief:

Ginger, citronella — stimulates tired feet

Basil, sandalwood — relaxes sore, aching feet

Citronella, bergamot — reduces excessive perspiration

Peppermint, lemon — soothes bunions

Ylang-ylang, lime — stimulates circulation from standing too long

Lemongrass, tea tree — antifungal and deodorising for athlete's foot

Ginger, eucalyptus, lemongrass, lemon — warming and invigorating for chilblains

Eucalyptus, ginger — revives and warms cold feet.

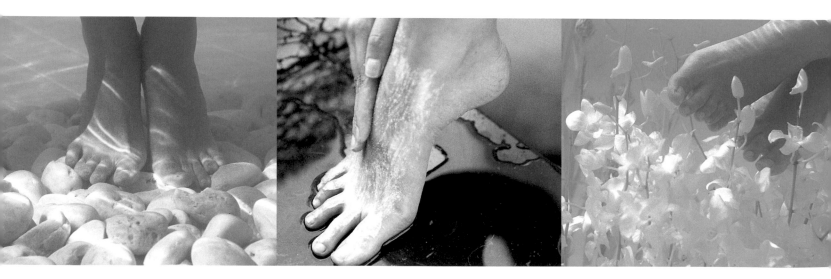

Sensuous Foot Soak

The Spa Botanica at the Sukhothai Bangkok recommends this soothing foot soak for tired feet, using the sensual, exotic scents of jasmine and sandalwood, two of the therapeutic trees that grow in the spa's lush, Thai-themed gardens.

2 cups	boiling water
1 cup	dried jasmine flowers
3–5 drops	sandalwood essential oil
1 cup	sea salt

Pour the hot water into a basin large enough to fit both feet. Add the jasmine flowers and salt, and let steep for 5–10 minutes. Add the sandalwood essential oil, and enough hot or cool water to cover your feet, and soak them for 10–15 minutes.

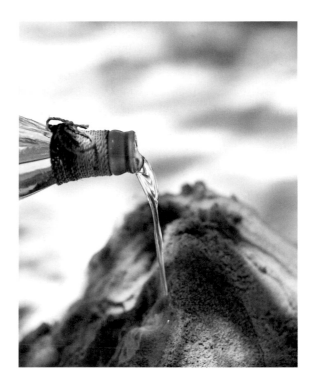

Beach Foot Polisher

An energetic walk on Thailand's soft, white sand beaches is one of the most natural therapies you can give yourself! Aside from exercising foot muscles that are normally restricted in shoes, sand has an exfoliating effect on the rough skin on your feet, and the soothing sensations of warm sea water ebbing and flowing between your toes is an added delight.

The Spa Botanica at the Sukhothai Bangkok tells you how to replicate that blissful beach mood while giving you the beauty benefits of the beach walk as well! This recipe uses beach sand as a natural exfoliant, and combines it with the richness of coconut oil as an emollient for skin that tends to be dry on the feet. Add either a few drops of peppermint essential oil to refresh and stimulate tired feet, or sandalwood essential oil to nourish feet that are rough or chapped.

3 tablespoons	fine beach sand
3 tablespoons	coconut oil
3–5 drops	sandalwood essential oil and/or
3–5 drops	peppermint essential oil

Mix all the ingredients together to make a paste. Massage the scrub onto your feet, gently exfoliating dead surface skin in the process. Rinse off with warm water and pat dry. This treatment feels extra good when followed with a warm foot bath.

Opposite, from left to right: Treading on rocks underwater massages the feet. Exfoliation is essential to foot care; try a cream like this peppermint scented foot scrub from Origins. An aromatherapy or floral foot soak is both relaxing and rejuvenating. *Above:* Coconut oil mixed with sand makes a moisturising foot scrub on the beach.

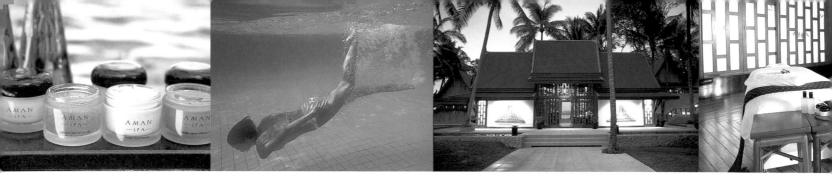

spa listings

Taking time out for a healing break at an exotic destination spa is one of the most rewarding treats you can give yourself. With its lush tropical landscape, palm-fringed beaches and islands, an abundance of succulent fruits and flowers, and delectable fresh and healthy cuisine, Thailand has become the top spa destination in Asia. Thailand's ancient traditions of herbal healing and traditional Thai massage are the sources of inspiration for the numerous spa concepts and treatments that abound in modern-day Thai spas. But the magical element that makes the Thai spa experience so alluring is that extra-special human touch — the sweet, sincere warmth of the Thai people and the gentle, caring spirit fostering a genuine pampering experience — that keeps visitors returning to Thailand again and again. Relaxing at a spa in Thailand is the ultimate retreat! Here we give you a list of the country's top luxury destination spas.

luxury destination spas in thailand

Aman Spa,
Amanpuri Resort, Phuket
P.O. Box 196, Pansea Beach
Phuket 83000
Tel: (66) 76 324 333
Fax: (66) 76 324 100 / 200
Email: amanpuri@amanresorts.com
Website: www.amanresorts.com

Angsana Spa Dusit Laguna Phuket
390 Srisoonthorn Road
Cherngtalay, Talang
Phuket 83110
Tel: (66) 76 324 320
Fax: (66) 76 324 174
Email: spa-dusitphuket@angsana.com
Website: www.angsana.com

Angsana Spa Green View Chiangmai
183/1 Chatana Road
Mae Sa-Mae Rim
Chiangmai 50180
Tel: (66) 53 298 249
Fax: (66) 53 297 386
Email: Spa-greenviewchiangmai
@angsana.com
Website: www.angsana.com

Angsana Spa Laguna Beach Resort
Phuket
323/2 Moo 2, Srisoonthorn Road
Cherngtalay, Talang, Phuket 83110
Tel: (66) 76 325 405
Fax: (66) 76 325 407
Email: spa-lagunabeachphuket
@angsana.com
Website: www.angsana.com

Angsana Spa Sheraton Grande
Laguna Beach Resort Phuket
10 Moo 4, Srisooonthorn Road
Cherngtalay, Talang
Phuket 83110
Tel: (66) 76 324 101
Fax: (66) 76 324 368
Email: spa-sheratonphuket
@angsana.com
Website: www.angsana.com

Banyan Tree Spa, Bangkok
21/100 South Sathon Road
Bangkok 10120
Tel: (66) 02 679 1200
Fax: (66) 02 673 1053
Email: spa-bangkok@banyantree.com
Website: www.banyantree.com

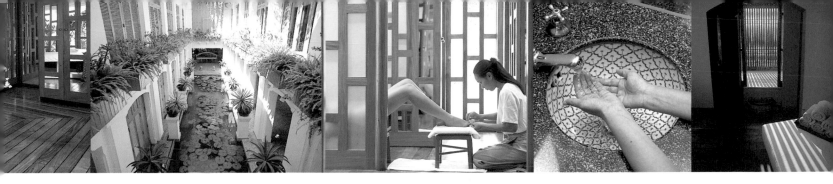

Banyan Tree Spa, Phuket
33 Moo 4 Srisoonthorn Road
Cherngtalay, Amphur Talang
Phuket 83110
Tel: (66) 76 324 374
Fax: (66) 76 271 463
Email: spa-phuket@banyantree.com
Website: www.banyantree.com

**Centara Spa, Central Samui Beach
Resort, Koh Samui**
38/2 Moo 3, Bophut, Chaweng Beach
Koh Samui 84310
Tel: (66) 77 230 500
Fax: (66) 77 422 385
Email: censamui@samart.com
Website: www.centralhotelsresorts.com

Chiva-Som, Hua Hin
73/4 Petchkasem Road, Hua Hin
Prachuab Khirikham 77110
Tel : (66) 32 536 536
Fax : (66) 32 51 1154
Email: reservation@chivasom.com
Website: www.chivasom.com

**Devarana Spa,
Dusit Thani Hotel Bangkok**
946 Rama 4 Road, Bangkok 10500
Tel: (66) 02 636 3596
Fax: (66) 02 636 3597
Email: bangkok@devarana.com
Website: www.devarana.com

The Imperial Mandara Spa
The Imperial Queen's Park Hotel
199 Sukhumvit Soi 22
Bangkok 10110
Tel: (66) 02 261 9000
Fax: (66) 02 261 9481
Email: imperial@mandaraspa-asia.com
Website: www.imperialhotels.com

**Lanna Spa,
The Regent Chiangmai**
Mae Rim-Samoeng Old Road
Mae Rim,
Chiangmai 50180
Tel: (66) 53 298 181
Fax: (66) 53 298 189
Email: rcm.lannaspa@fourseasons.com
Website: www.regenthotels.com

**Le Royal Spa,
Le Royal Meridien Phuket Yacht Club**
Nai Harn Beach
Phuket 83130
Tel: (66) 76 380 200–19
Fax: (66) 76 380 280
Email: PYCrsvn@meridien.co.th
Website: www.phuket-yachtclub.com

**Mandara Spa,
Anantara Resort & Spa, Hua Hin**
43/1 Phetkasem Road
Hua Hin 77110
Tel: (66) 32 520 250
Fax: (66) 32 520 259
Email: anantara@mandaraspa-asia.com
Website: www.anantara.com

**Mandara Spa,
Bangkok Marriott Resort & Spa, Bkk**
257/1-3 Charoen Nakhon Road
At the Krungthep Bridge
Bangkok 10600
Tel: (66) 02 476 0021
Fax: (66) 02 476 1120
Email: bmrs@mandaraspa-asia.com
Website: www.marriotthotels.com/bkkth

**Mandara Spa,
Hua Hin Marriott Resort & Spa**
107/1 Phetkasem Beach Road,
Hua Hin 77110

Tel: (66) 32 511 882/4
Fax: (66) 32 512 422
Email: hmrs@mandaraspa-asia.com
Website: www.marriotthotels.com

**Mandara Spa,
JW Marriott Phuket Resort & Spa**
Moo 3, Mai Khao, Talang
Phuket 83140
Tel: (66) 76 33 8000
Fax: (66) 76 34 8348
Email: jwmp@mandaraspa-asia.com
Website: www.marriott.com and
www.phuket.com/marriott/

**The Oriental Spa,
The Oriental Bangkok**
48 Oriental Avenue, Bangkok
Tel: (66) 02 439 7613-4
Fax: (66) 02 439 7885
Email: orawanc@mohg.com
Website: www.mandarinoriental.com

**Santiburi Spa,
Santiburi Dusit Resort, Samui**
Santiburi Dusit Resort
12/12 Moo 1, Tambol Mae Nam
Koh Samui 84330
Tel: (66) 77 42 5031-8
Fax: (66) 77 42 5040
Email: santiburi@dusit.com
Website: www.dusit.com

**Spa Botanica,
The Sukhothai Bangkok
(*opening in 2003)**
13/3 Sathorn Road
Bangkok 10120
Tel: (66) 02 287 0222
Fax: (66) 02 287 4980 / 285 0133
Email: info@sukhothai.com
Website: www.sukhothai.com

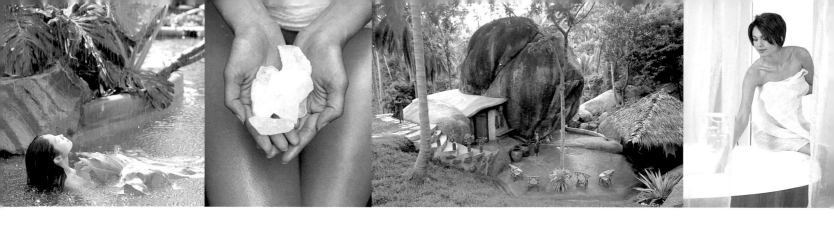

thai traditional herbal day spas

Not all spas are destination resorts. Thailand offers a number of charming boutique day spas around the country. The following day spas specialise in traditional Thai healing therapies, and offer a range of ancient herbal healing treatments and traditional massage, along with modern-day spa treatments. Though not in the luxury range, these spas offer a cosy atmosphere in attractive environments, and are conveniently located and priced, for a spot of quick pampering whether you are a visitor or resident in Thailand.

Ban Sabai Spa, Chiangmai
17/7 Chalerm Prathet Road
Near Night Bazaar
Chiangmai 50100
Tel: (66) 53 285 204-6
Fax: (66) 53 270 468
Email: info@ban-sabai.com
Website: www.ban-sabai.com

Ban Sabai Spa, Koh Samui
59 Moo 4, Bophut, Bangrak
Big Buddha Beach
Samui 84320
Tel: (66) 77 245 175, 77 427 444
Fax: (66) 77 245 176
Email: info@ban-sabai.com
Website: www.ban-sabai.com

Nakriya House of Health & Beauty, Bangkok
31/6 Soi Promjai, Sukhumvit Soi 39
Bangkok 10110
Tel: (66) 02 260 6295-6
Fax: (66) 02 662 2718
Email: none
Website: none

Palm Herbal Spa, Bangkok
103 Soi Thonglor
17 Sukhumvit 55 Road
Bangkok 10110
Tel / Fax: (66) 02 391 3153
Email: palmherbal2002@hotmail.com
Website: www.palmherbalspa.com

Thai Herbal Spa, Bangkok
10th Floor,
Waterford Diamond Tower
758/14 Sukhumvit Soi 30/1
Bangkok 10110
Tel: (66) 02 665 6550-1 ext. 1001, 1002
Fax: (66) 02 261 6263
Email: none
Website: none

Tamarind Retreat, Koh Samui
205/7 Moo 4, Thong Takian
Tambol Maret
Koh Samui 84310
Tel: (66) 77 230 571
Fax: (66) 77 424 311
Email: info@tamarindretreat.com
Website: www.tamarindretreat.com

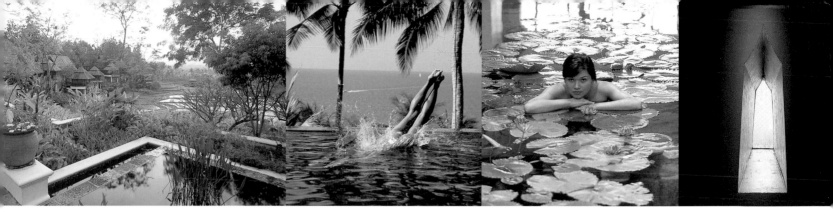

acknowledgments

We would like to thank many people who gave their kind assistance during the production of this book. In particular, the author would like to express special thanks to Mr Ian Bell of the Aman Spa at the Amanpuri Resort, for his thoughtful contributions and generous support during the writing of this book. Special thanks also go to Khun Komon Chitprasert of the Thai Herbal Spa, Bangkok, who shared his valuable knowledge on traditional medicine and ancient herbal lore.

We would like to express our deepest thanks to Ms Trina Dingler Ebert of Aman Resorts, Ms Liv Gussing of the Amanpuri Resort, Ms Reene Ho-Phang of Banyan Tree Hotels & Resorts, Khun Sirima Eamtako of the Banyan Tree and Angsana Spas Phuket, Ms Jennifer Ng-Lim and Ms Miriam van Doorn of the Spa Botanica, Khun Susie Hansirisawasdi and Khun Anuttra Chinalai of the Oriental Bangkok, Khun Orawan Choeysawat of the Oriental Spa, Mr Jens Reichert and Ms Monica Orias of Mandara Spa, Ms Kymberley Sproule of the Regent Chiangmai Resort, Khun Rungratree Kongkwanyuen of the Lanna Spa at the Regent Chiangmai, Ms Belinda Shepherd of the Four Seasons Resorts, Mr Olivier Gibaud of Le Royal Meridien Phuket Yacht Club, Khun Narumol Sukapojana of Le Royal Spa, at Le Royal Meridien Phuket Yacht Club, Ms Shelley Poplak of Tamarind Retreat, Khun Wipawadee Sirimongkolkasem of the Dusit Group, Khun Shelida Buranasiri of Nakriya House of Health & Beauty, Mae-Chee Sansanee of Sathira-Dhammasthan Ashram, Mr Albert Paravi Wongchirachai, Mr Bill Bensley, Mr Eugene Davis, Khun Teddy Spha Palasthira, the von Buerens of Lotus Arts de Vivre, Khun Dee Dee of Goods Goods Koh Samui, Khun Worapan Opapan of Origins, Khun Vipawadee Thangkitpithakpol, Khun Nagara Sambandaraksa, Mr Jean-Michel and Khun Patsri Beurdeley.

Also many thanks to our bevy of beautiful models:
Sirinya Burbridge (Cindy)
Kunlanut Pieyawat (Nam Fon)
Methinee Kingpayom (Kathy)
Sonia Couling
Helen Berger
Haley Berger (baby)
Rai von Bueren
Janice Nopvichai
Chalitda Panitchakarn (Maew)
Varalux Vanichkul (Joy)
Niki Frei

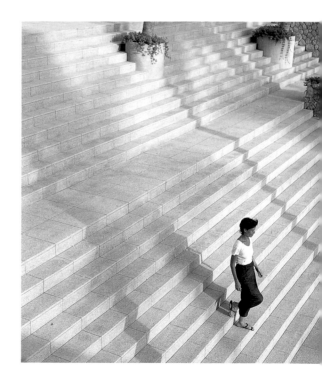

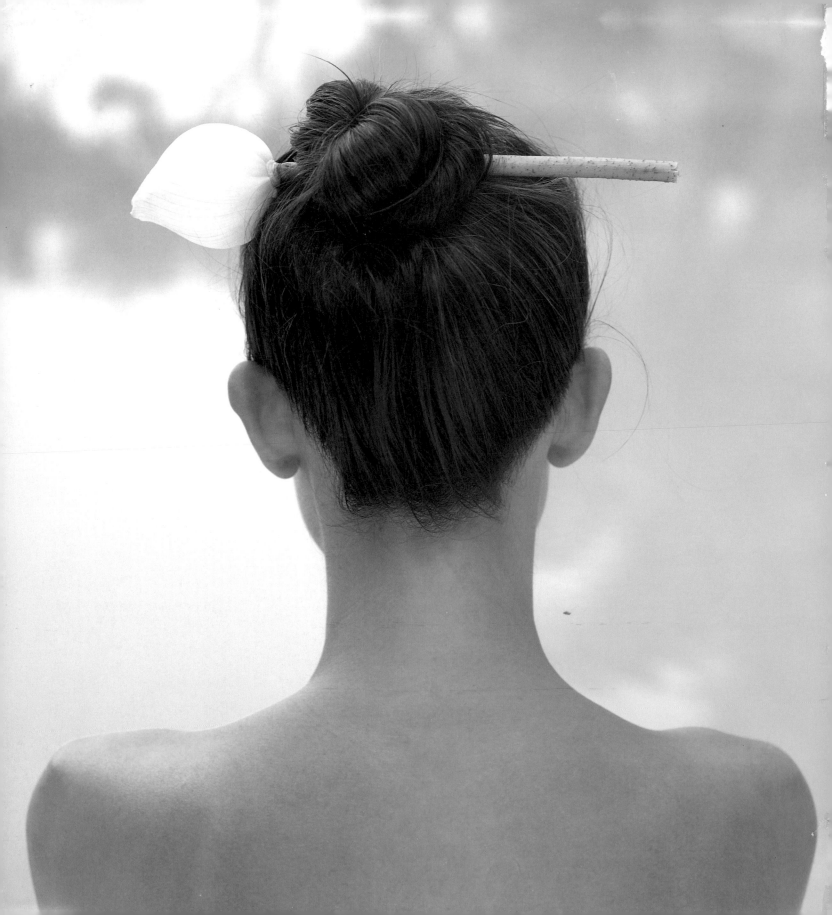